# IVF Meal Plan

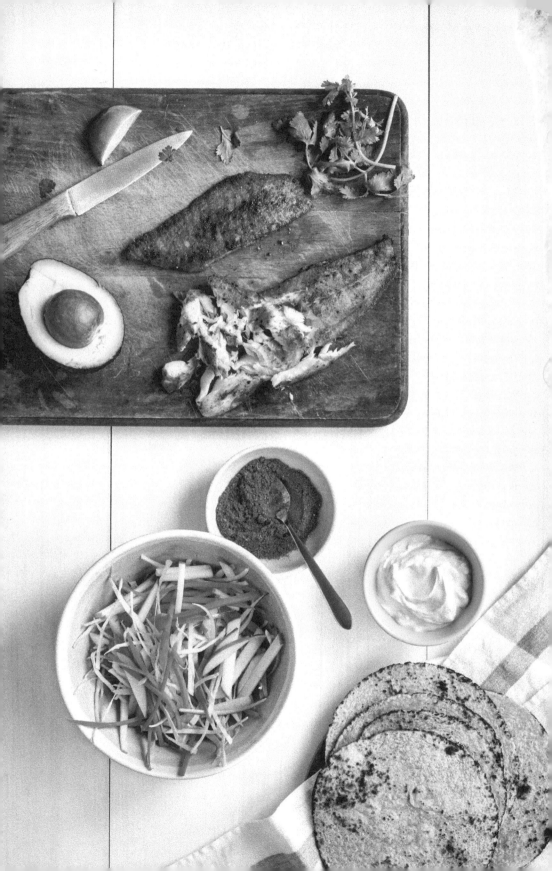

# IVF MEAL PLAN

Maximize Your Chances of
IVF Success Through Diet

Dr. Elizabeth Cherevaty, ND, RAC

ROCKRIDGE
PRESS

*For the next generation*

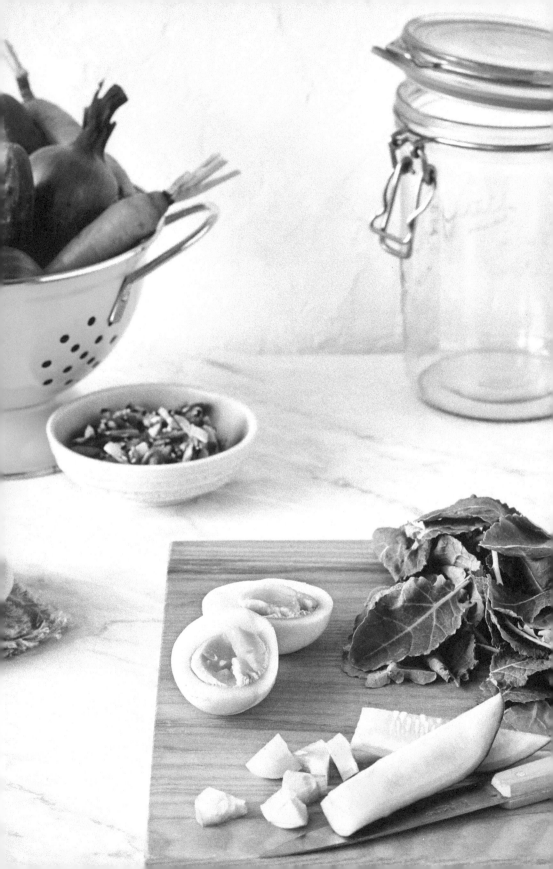

# CONTENTS

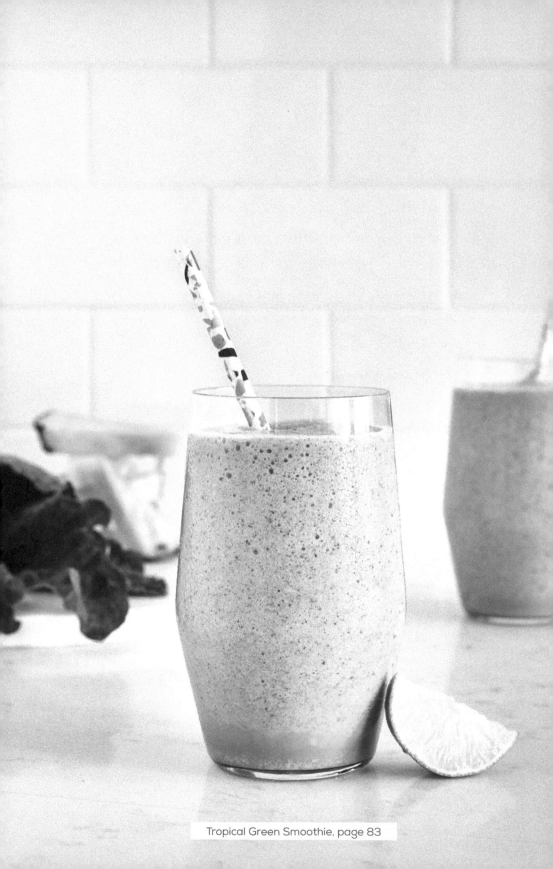

Tropical Green Smoothie, page 83

# INTRODUCTION

For some, conception happens easily, even without thought; for others, it becomes an all-consuming challenge that often feels out of their control.

Although some factors affecting fertility are beyond our control, plenty more are well within our ability to alter and reverse. Throughout this book, you'll learn about powerful external factors—such as specific foods and lifestyle changes—that fertility researchers have found can affect not only conception, but also egg quality and fetal health. These factors can also affect the long-term health and even the reproductive success of our offspring.

During my naturopathic internship, I worked with kids who suffered from chronic health problems—from feeding and digestive issues, to eczema, allergies, and asthma, to behavior and learning challenges—at ages much younger than the textbooks suggested were "normal." I was alarmed to learn that, for the first time in history, a generation of children was not expected to outlive their parents. Yet, around the same time of my internship, newly published research showed that at least some risk factors for certain chronic diseases were preventable—especially with improved pregnancy and childbirth.

Inspired by the potential to prevent certain fertility troubles as well as a traditional Chinese medicine practice in which couples consciously devote a "season" to enhancing their own well-being *before they conceive* in order to give their future baby the greatest possible health "inheritance," I expanded my clinical focus to include preconception. I opened my own integrative and naturopathic family care practice, Two Rivers Health, and created the Well Conceived Fertility Method™ to help forge a healthier path from preconception to pediatrics for future generations. Well Conceived™ equips couples with evidence-based strategies to reverse the effects of modern life's health and fertility pressures (such as environmental pollution, processed food, sedentary lifestyles, and endless stress). These strategies not only help them conceive, but also help them invest in their future children's health. They are based on *epigenetics*—the study of the influence of environmental factors and lifestyle choices (such as diet) on the genetic expression of descendants.

I once consulted with a fertility specialist on behalf of a patient who was discharged from her previous IVF clinic with a diagnosis of "poor egg quality." The patient had seen some positive changes in our work together, and I wanted to know whether, if we continued on the path of targeted food and lifestyle tweaks, she might be reassessed and considered a good candidate to try IVF again. He said, "There's nothing *we* can do about egg quality . . . but there are things *she* can do."

It sounds too good to be true, but our food *communicates* with our genes. Have you ever had a friend who came home from a great vacation, started a new exercise plan, or finally left a stressful relationship, and suddenly looked 10 years younger? That's the power of epigenetics at work: same genes, different environmental influences! Why not get your food "talking" to your genes in a way that benefits your fertility? The recipes in this book, developed by chef and educator Charleston F. Dollano, will help you do just that.

Over the next few months, we're going to put one of the guiding principles of naturopathic medical practice—"food as medicine"—to work for you. Although eating a healthy diet is important to fertility and overall health, research shows that not every "healthy diet" is a "fertility diet." In this book, I'll show you why certain foods impact fertility and IVF success rates and give you an easy-to-follow map to success.

Bring your partner along for the ride. The changes you'll be making will benefit your partner's fertility and health, too. You two are on the path to parenthood together.

Whether you've been trying to get pregnant for a long time or you're just starting to consider IVF, I want you to know that *transformation is possible*. It's not about wishing, it's about nourishing your body, mind, and fertility with an evidence-based plan. I've seen it work for countless couples who have come through our clinic seeking a miracle, and I'm excited to help you experience your miracle, too.

## SETTING YOURSELF UP FOR SUCCESS

As an egg (*oocyte*) is being prepared for ovulation—or for retrieval in an IVF cycle—maturation of the follicle that nourishes it is governed by hormones. Depending on your situation, you may be able to promote that maturation during the wait time before your IVF cycle actually begins. Ask your integrative fertility practitioner to test for nutrients such as iron, vitamin $B_{12}$, vitamin D, and folate. Also ask to be examined for pregnancy risk factors such as high homocysteine, blood sugar, or autoimmunity markers and find out whether a more detailed hormone or genomics panel would be helpful for you as you prepare for IVF.

# OMG POAS BFP IVF: DECODING THE LANGUAGE

Acronym overwhelm, be gone! This book's glossary of common medical abbreviations (page 155) will come in handy throughout your IVF journey, but it won't necessarily help you decipher the shorthand language found in online fertility forums. Here are the most popular informal IVF acronyms:

**2WW:** "two-week wait" between ovulation or IVF transfer and testing for pregnancy

**AF:** "Aunt Flo," menstruation

**Baby Dust:** a wish for good (fertility) luck

**Beta:** beta-hCG, the hormone detected in a pregnancy test; also refers to the hormone estradiol

**BD:** "baby dance," sexual intercourse

**BFN:** "big fat negative," a negative pregnancy test

**BFP:** "big fat positive," a positive pregnancy test

**CF, CM:** cervical fluid/mucus

**CP:** cervical position

**DH:** "dear husband" or **DW:** "dear wife"

**DTD:** "do/did the deed," have/had sexual intercourse

**EWCM:** egg white cervical mucus

**FF, FM:** fertile fluid/mucus

**Frostie:** frozen embryo

**FTTA:** "fertile thoughts to all"

**HPT:** home pregnancy test

**IB:** implantation bleeding

**Line eyes:** asking for others to consider whether an OPK or HPT is positive or negative

**MENTS:** "my exciting news to share"

**OMG:** "Oh my God!"

**OPK, OPT:** ovulation predictor kit/test

**POAS:** "pee on a stick"

**Rainbow baby:** a baby born after the loss of a pregnancy or child

**Sensitive:** material may be difficult for others to see/read

**WYOO:** "What's your opinion on . . ."

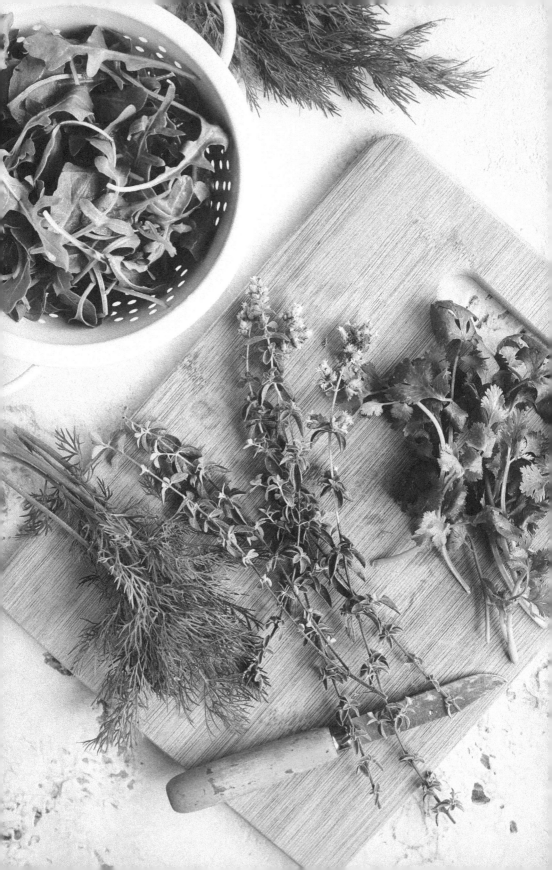

# PART ONE

# Everything You Need to Know About How Food Impacts Your Egg Quality

Blackened Fish Tacos, page 99

# CHAPTER ONE

# The Intersection of Egg Quality and Diet

Have you ever heard that the human body completely regenerates itself every seven years? When I was about six years old, a friend shared this astounding news with me. I couldn't wait to wake up on my seventh birthday to discover a brand-new body! Although our bodies don't transform overnight as my childhood brain imagined, they are in a continuous state of renewal.

Cells have a predefined life span, before the end of which most will copy and replace themselves. The building blocks for creating and maintaining new cells come from the food we eat. That's why our food has a direct and almost immediate effect on our health—and therefore on our fertility. When we choose foods that provide the highest-quality materials for healthy new cells, we set the foundation for our fertility to flourish. And because every system of the body benefits from nutritious food, we feel more energized overall.

# What Does Food Have to Do with IVF?

According to a study published in the scientific journal *Fertility and Sterility*, consumption of nutritious foods during preconception can increase a couple's chances of IVF pregnancy by as much as 40 percent. In the months before you ovulate or have your egg retrieval for IVF, the food you eat influences your fertility through nutritional and hormonal factors.

Although your complete reproductive lifetime's supply of eggs has been in your ovaries since your birth, they've essentially been in a state of suspended animation. About three months before ovulation, specific hormonal signals recruit a follicle (the nourishing sac containing the egg) to enter its final stage of development, during which the egg is nurtured and prepared for ovulation. During this three-month preconception window, your diet helps ensure that ample nutrients are invested in follicle growth and egg maturation and that specific nutrients like antioxidants protect the egg (and the DNA within it) from potential damage induced by environmental toxins and usual cellular metabolism. In fact, according to an article published in *Trends in Genetics*, the stage just before ovulation is one of the most vulnerable times for chromosomal abnormalities to occur. Your diet will either promote regulation or dysregulation of a fertility-friendly hormonal balance, especially through the stimulation of insulin, which influences levels of other hormones. Ensuring that your diet is nutrient rich and hormone healthy is a powerful strategy to support your chances of having a successful IVF cycle and a healthy baby.

# Eating for Three
# (You and Your Ovaries)

Micronutrient malnutrition—inadequate intake of vitamins, minerals, and antioxidants—is common in both developed and developing countries. Fertility-specific results of malnutrition include incomplete stores of building blocks needed for DNA synthesis and repair, hormonal imbalances that inhibit follicle maturation, and increased levels of inflammation. All of these phenomena create cell and DNA damage and may alter the hospitality of the pregnancy environment.

In 2013, a study published in the journal *Human Reproduction Update* brought to light a key area of fertility-specific malnutrition called one-carbon (1-C) metabolism. The role of 1-C metabolism is to deliver "methyl" groups—seemingly simple molecules with one carbon and three hydrogen atoms, or $CH_3$—which play a critical role in the synthesis of DNA. Deficiency of micronutrients, specifically methionine, vitamin $B_{12}$, and folate, during the critical preconception period of oocyte growth and fertilization—as well as up to the first 10 weeks of pregnancy—contributes to the risk of miscarriage and long-term health problems in children. You may be familiar with how adequate dietary folic acid (folate) intake can prevent neural tube defects. This is an example of 1-C metabolism at work. More broadly, normal genetic variations, such as having genes that code for enzymes that either increase or decrease the speed of certain steps of our metabolism, combined with malnutrition, may upset 1-C metabolism in ways that are harmful to egg quality, embryo competence, pregnancy success, and even the health of the next generation.

Modern malnutrition in developed countries is demonstrated by overnutrition in terms of calories (especially sugars or carbohydrates) and undernutrition in terms of micronutrients (including vitamins, minerals, omega-3 fats, and antioxidants). This nutritional imbalance perpetuates hormonal dysregulation and inflammation and compromises the health potential of eggs, embryos, and even future babies. The good news is, you are capable of easily fixing this issue as it pertains to your own body. In chapter 2, we'll take a closer look at how to reverse this pattern and prepare yourself for a fertility-friendly diet.

## Your Ovaries Are Actually Geniuses

About 24 weeks before ovulation, a hormone signals the ovary to stimulate development of five to seven follicles. Follicular development is most intensive during the 12 weeks before ovulation and the release of an egg from one "dominant" follicle. (In an IVF cycle, medications are given to increase the number of follicles that develop, so multiple eggs can be retrieved for intended fertilization.)

To be viable, embryos need a normal number of intact chromosomes. Half of these chromosomes come from the egg, and the other half come from sperm. IVF success rates decline as women age because of increased frequency of chromosomal misalignments and increased levels of oxidative stress to the chromosomes.

Chromosomally speaking, egg quality can be affected in any of three key biological stages: The first two stages occur in utero during a female's fetal life. The third stage is during the three to six months before you conceive. During the final stage of follicular development, the DNA within the egg resumes chromosomal division. The correct division of chromosomes is dependent on a full supply of energy from the egg's mitochondria as well as on adequate protection against DNA-damaging toxins and oxidative stress. (The corresponding sensitive time for sperm is during spermatogenesis—the process of sperm cell production.)

Thus, as your eggs are completing their final countdown to launch, you have an opportunity to make a nutritional investment in your fertility and pregnancy success as well as in your child's future health. Your health-supportive diet will supply required nutrients, positively influence hormonal health, provide protection from environmental toxins, and boost mitochondrial function to give your eggs the best possible chances to avoid chromosomal abnormalities. That's a lot of power.

When you follow the meal plans provided in this book, you will be supporting egg health and follicle quality in order to:

- ▼ Enhance the supply of nutrients that enrich eggs, follicles, and DNA and protect them from damage
- ▼ Reduce inflammation, which is a key cause of oxidative stress and DNA damage
- ▼ Improve hormone health in ways that aid egg development
- ▼ Reduce the intake and impact of environmental toxins
- ▼ Prepare the body for a healthy pregnancy and a healthy baby

## Take a Deep Breath, and Make Up with Your Body

Fertility challenges can trigger a full range of painful emotions. The fertility journey affects every aspect of your life's vision: your relationship, family, self-worth, and sense of purpose. If you've felt betrayed by your own body or resentful or frustrated that pregnancy isn't coming easily for you or harbored a sense of failure or shame that you haven't been able to have a baby, you're not alone. These feelings are a natural response to very difficult circumstances, and getting the right supports in place is important to release these emotions so they won't linger and create additional suffering and ultimately affect your health and fertility goals.

While establishing your foundation of good nutrition, devote efforts to nourishing yourself in every way. Invite a loving relationship between yourself and your body. When you get your period, think of it as a stage of renewal. Your body is working hard to nurture the eggs that are waiting in the wings, and it will recruit the best follicles to groom for the next opportunity for conception. Think of these soon-to-be developed eggs as young recruits, and give them all the encouragement you can. Keep in mind that every period is one cycle closer to your next opportunity to conceive.

From a place of deep self-connection, you'll be better equipped to calm hormonal chaos caused by high levels of cortisol, you'll feel at greater peace with what your body is communicating through the stages of your menstrual cycles, and you'll feel more in control as you prepare for IVF.

# Common Health Conditions and Fertility

Unrecognized health conditions can affect fertility, so it's worth a discussion with your doctor to ensure that any potential underlying contributors to fertility challenges have been properly addressed or ruled out. Here are four of the most common health issues that can make it difficult to conceive.

## Autoimmune Conditions

"Autoimmunity" refers to the response of one's own immune system to attack some aspect of the body through the production and action of proteins produced by the immune system, called antibodies. Several fertility-related conditions, including endometriosis and premature ovarian failure, involve autoimmune mechanisms, and autoimmunity is a risk factor for miscarriage. According to a 2019 review published in the *International Journal of Molecular Sciences*, autoimmunity is a possible "explanation" for unexplained infertility and there may be links between autoimmunity and premature ovarian failure, recurrent miscarriage, and IVF failure.

The majority of thyroid conditions are caused by autoimmunity. With Hashimoto's disease, the immune system produces antibodies that bind with certain components of thyroid hormone production or function. A systematic review published in *Human Reproductive Update* in 2011 associated thyroid autoimmunity with increased odds of having unexplained infertility, 3.73-times greater odds of having a miscarriage, and 1.9-times greater odds of premature birth. In a 2014 study of women with Graves' disease (another type of thyroid autoimmunity) and Hashimoto's thyroiditis, 52 percent and 47 percent of women with these disorders, respectively, also had infertility.

Thyroid autoimmunity is assessed through blood work. Successful treatment may include a combination of diet, herbal, and supplement therapies, and/or prescription thyroid hormone replacement.

Celiac disease is caused by an autoimmune attack on the inner lining of the intestinal tract, leading to inflammation and lack of absorption of important nutrients that are required to support fertility and health. Testing for celiac disease may involve blood work and an intestinal biopsy. Celiac's auto-immune attack on the gut can be halted by eliminating gluten (found in the grains wheat, rye, barley, triticale, spelt, and kamut) from the diet.

## Gum Health

As distant from the reproductive system as the mouth is, there may be a connection between both men's and women's oral health and their fertility. A 2017 review in the *Journal of Obstetrics and Gynecology of India* noted associations between the presence of gingivitis—a low-grade inflammation or infection hidden in the gums—and poor sperm quality, reduced chances of natural and IVF conception, and increased risk of pregnancy complications. The bacteria from gingi-vitis can enter the bloodstream to affect distant tissues and increase inflammation in the body as a whole. It can't hurt to ensure that you and your partner are both up to date with your dental checkups.

## Stress

It's not just "in your head." Studies show that preconception stress in either partner can increase the risk of stress-related disorders for a couple's future children. Stress and trauma cause changes in microRNA that impact genetic expression and proteins necessary for positive mental health and resiliency. These changes have been shown to affect two or more generations! We know that the stress of trying to get pregnant can be intense. It doesn't feel good, and through epigenetic programming it can affect your future child and even your child's future child. Stress can affect hormone levels, including DHEA, a hormone that's important for maintaining egg quality. In a 1998 study published in the journal *Integrative Psychological and Behavioral Science*, participants were taught to use negative thought–interrupting techniques to create a low-stress, positive emotional state compellingly named "warmheartedness," which was found to be associated with higher DHEA and lower cortisol levels. Thought loops tend to be persistent, triggering painful emotions until we take notice and take charge of our "self-talk."

Use your thoughts to be kind to yourself. Take loving care of yourself during this time. Getting support if you feel anxious, depressed, tense, tearful, or irritable will help you and your partner though this challenging time, and will benefit your hormone health, your personal experience, and your baby's future mental and emotional wellness. Win-win-win.

## Digestive Health

As the source of general food sensitivities, diagnosed food intolerances, and other conditions like irritable bowel syndrome (IBS), the digestive tract is a critical interface between our external and internal environments. Unless food is efficiently digested by stomach acid, intestinal enzymes, and bile fluid and then absorbed through our intestines, we can't benefit from its nutritional content. I've found in my practice that digestive disturbances and food sensitivities are common and often undertreated. These issues increase inflammation in the body, may trigger inappropriate immunological responses, and can make toxin elimination less efficient. Digestive problems also compromise the body's ability to absorb nutrients that are important to your fertility and baby's development, including iron, vitamin $B_{12}$, and vitamin D. If you have digestive symptoms such as loose stools or constipation, abdominal pain or cramping associated with meals, gas or bloating, or have taken antibiotics, you'll most likely benefit from some healing and optimizing of your digestive system.

# YOU'RE OFF THE HOOK FOR THREE MONTHS

Are you ready to take a break from the many pressures that come with trying to get pregnant?

First, if charting has been stressful, let me clarify for you the two most valuable indicators to track: cervical fluid (CF) and basal body temperature (BBT). These two may be worth tracking even as you prepare for IVF because they'll provide information you and your integrative fertility practitioner can use to refine your IVF prep plan. Unless you're trying to conceive naturally, consider hitting pause on ovulation prediction kits. They only predict, but can't confirm, ovulation.

Next, consider whether it's time to take a break from self-prescribed supplements. (We'll look more at the science behind egg health–specific supplements in chapter 3.) Remember that, as strong as their safety profiles may be, supplements are in fact medicines and should be treated as such, especially in light of the high-stakes goals of getting pregnant and having a healthy baby. For example, Canadian regulation of "natural health products" (NHPs) is among the most stringent in the world, but supplements are regulated differently in the United States and other countries, which can mean consumers are basically left to their own devices. See the resources section (page 161) for tips on sourcing safe, condition-specific NHPs. Before choosing any supplements, consult with a licensed health practitioner experienced in integrative fertility care, who can make sure that any NHPs you choose to take are right for you at this stage.

Finally, here's a golden opportunity to take the pressure out of the bedroom. Set aside time when you can be alone and reconnect as a couple. Eliminating the pressure to perform will make it easier to enjoy your relationship, and you may find your desire for intimacy increases when you're both relaxed and "off the clock."

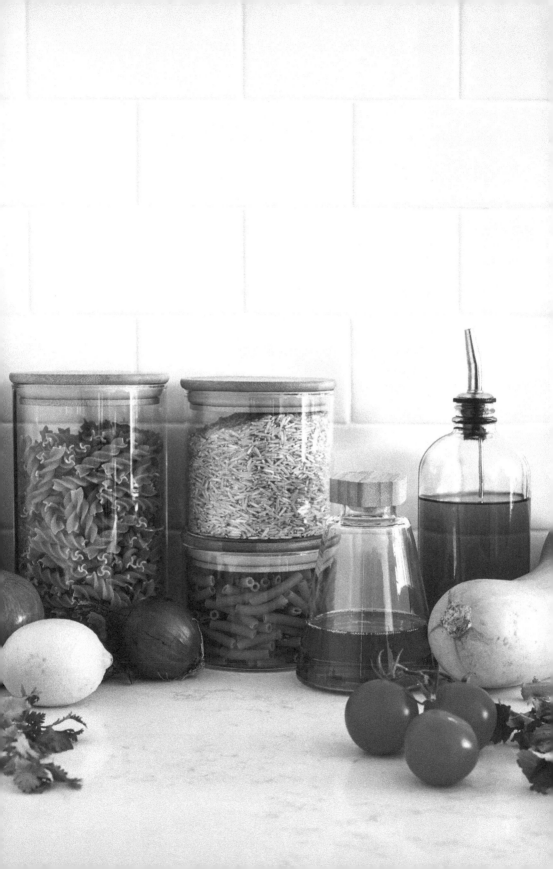

# CHAPTER TWO

# Preparing for
# the Meal Plan

Hundreds of studies now point to the presence of harmful industrial chemicals in air, soil, water, plants, and animal tissues. At the top of the food chain, we humans consume all of the above, and so our bodies contain measurable levels of these contaminants. Diet is the first line of defense against these toxins, second only to your everyday habits at home.

As a naturopathic doctor with a premedical degree in toxicology, I've had many conversations about toxins and fertility with clients in my clinic and online courses. From the diverse potential avenues we could explore, I've whittled the list down to the two most important strategies to minimize the havoc environmental toxins can wreak on fertility: reduce exposure and enrich your diet (food and supplements) with the nutrients required for your body's innate detoxification systems to function.

Let's tackle exposure reduction, from table to toiletries!

# Make Your Kitchen Fertility Friendly

When it comes to the kitchen and grocery shopping, you have two objectives as you prepare for your IVF meal plans: get rid of anything processed, and choose products in non-plastic packaging whenever possible. Following is a detailed list of fertility-friendly kitchen swap-ins as well as some important information about bisphenol A (BPA), a chemical commonly found in plastics.

## Pitch Processed Foods

Processed foods undergo intensive mechanical or chemical processes to convert them into the forms we see on the grocery store shelf, and as such, they are likely to be a source of toxins and a trigger of inflammation and hormone havoc. Time to show these common offenders where to go, John Wayne–style: Let's head 'em up and move 'em out.

| | REMOVE FROM YOUR KITCHEN | ENJOY INSTEAD |
|---|---|---|
| **FATS AND OILS** | Cooking spray<br>Corn oil<br>Margarine<br>Palm oil<br>Peanut oil<br>Shortening<br>Soy oil<br>Vegetable oil | **FOR HIGH-HEAT COOKING**<br>Avocado oil<br>Butter (organic/pasture-raised/grass-fed cows)<br>Coconut oil<br>Grapeseed oil<br>Tallow |
| | | **TO EAT RAW OR DRIZZLED OVER COOKED FOOD**<br>Extra-virgin olive oil<br>Flaxseed oil<br>Walnut oil |

| | REMOVE FROM YOUR KITCHEN | ENJOY INSTEAD |
|---|---|---|
| **FOOD ADDITIVES** | Alcohol and caffeine | Blackstrap molasses |
| | Artificial sweeteners such as aspartame, sucralose, cyclamate, acesulfame-K, saccharin | Date sugar |
| | | Erythritol |
| | | Honey |
| | | Maple syrup |
| | | Xylitol |
| | Food colorings such as "FD&C" dyes, colored frosting and syrups | |
| | Preservatives such as sodium benzoate, tartrazine, polysorbate | |
| | Stevia | |
| **CARBO-HYDRATES** | Candy | Fruits and vegetables |
| | Refined sugar, such as white sugar, brown sugar, dextrose, glucose, glucose-fructose, high-fructose corn syrup, corn syrup solids, table syrup | Grain-free starches such as potatoes, squash, carrots, parsnips, turnips, beets, yams |
| | Sodas and sweetened beverages | Whole grains such as brown rice, quinoa, millet, oatmeal |
| | White flour breads, crackers, baked goods, pastries, all-purpose flour, noodles | Whole-grain breads, pastas, crackers, etc. |

## Purge Plastics

When our food and beverages come into contact with plastics, they leach endocrine disruptors, chemicals that disrupt hormone health, fertility, and even fetal development. Among the most prevalent are bisphenol A (BPA) and phthalates.

A 2019 study published in the *International Journal of Endocrinology* found that BPA disrupts fertility by mimicking estrogen, interfering with androgens, impairing thyroid function, and reducing follicle counts in women. BPA is detectable in follicular fluid, where it comes into direct contact with oocytes and can disrupt follicle maturation and increase chromosomal abnormalities. A 2010 study published in the *International Journal of Andrology* found that women with higher concentrations of BPA in their urine had lower numbers of eggs retrieved during their IVF cycles.

BPA exposure also negatively impacts sperm quality and male fertility. One report published in the journal *Reproductive Toxicology* noted that *prenatal* exposure to BPA may be the most concerning, due to its negative affects on developing fetal endocrine systems and brains. Furthermore, various scientific studies have highlighted the harmful associations of prenatal BPA exposure on children's future health outcomes, from asthma to neurobehavioral issues.

It sounds scary, but the good news is that you can make a tremendous impact on your BPA exposure. Simply put, reducing BPA exposure starts in the grocery store. As much as possible, purchase prepared foods like oils, salad dressings, spreads, and nut butters in non-plastic containers, such as glass jars. Even some canned goods leach BPA from the coating that lines the can. Choose BPA-free cans, always rinse canned foods before using them, or choose fresh or dried versions with plastic-free packaging whenever possible. Replace plastic food and beverage storage containers and equipment with fertility-safe alternatives like waxed paper and glass, bamboo, silicone, or stainless steel containers and equipment. Use a carbon filter or reverse osmosis system to filter and dispense tap water (see Resources, page 161). Even plastics marked BPA-free may contain other bisphenols that may prove equally problematic, so choose plastic-free for anything that comes into contact with food or beverages whenever possible.

At home, choose cast iron, enamel, glass, or stainless-steel cookware. Never microwave with plastics, and toss any plastics that have been heated, run through the dishwasher, or left out in the car. Worn-down plastics leach the highest concentrations of toxic chemicals into food and beverages stored or prepared in them, so now's the time to get rid of them, too.

## Make Your Bathroom Fertility Friendly

Our next stop on this fertility-friendly cleansing train: toiletries. A recent report by the Environmental Working Group (EWG) indicated that the average American woman is exposed to 168 different toxic chemicals before even leaving the house in the morning. Several of these chemicals have been shown to disrupt hormones, decrease fertility, or harm fetal development—no, thank you!

Read on to learn how to eliminate many of these hidden villains from your daily routine.

### Phthalates

One of the EWG's "Dirty Dozen Endocrine Disruptors" (2013), phthalates are hidden in an estimated 75 percent of personal care products, as components of "fragrance," "parfum," or "perfume." Phthalates trigger testicular cell death, sperm abnormalities, and male reproductive system defects with prenatal exposure. They've also been associated with the development of diabetes, obesity, and thyroid issues.

Current cosmetics regulations in both the United States and Canada do not require manufacturers to list the ingredients that make up a fragrance on product labels, so the best way to avoid these toxins is to go fragrance-free. Being both aware of the hidden toxicity of fragrances and particularly sensitive to scents, I don't feel well when I'm around even a whiff of synthetic fragrance, so I asked family members not to wear perfume or cologne to family events and get-togethers. Although it felt a bit awkward at first to impose a no-fragrance policy on my loved ones, now everyone happily obliges, and I get to feel happy at Thanksgiving and merry at Christmas!

Phthalates are also found in plastics with a "3" or higher recycling symbol, which is another good reason to purge plastics from your lifestyle.

## Parabens

Parabens are a family of compounds that are added to cosmetics as preservatives. They're easier to spot on product labels by the suffix *paraben*—as in propylparaben, methylparaben, and butylparaben. Look for these chemicals on product labels, particularly those of cream- or lotion-based products like sunscreens and moisturizers, and steer clear. Parabens are problematic because they mimic estrogen.

A recent review published in *Physiological Research* observed that parabens may also compromise the body's ability to detoxify BPA, making them of even greater concern for preconception and prenatal exposure.

## Pesticides

Any product that contains non-organic plant ingredients may be contaminated with traces of pesticides, which, of course, won't be listed on labels. Many pesticides can dissolve through the skin into the bloodstream, so I prefer organic personal care products during preconception and pregnancy, and for newborns and kids of all ages.

# Prescription Drugs and OTCs

Several types of prescription drugs affect fertility and/or pregnancy. This isn't an exhaustive list—just a few key categories of common medications that you should know about. Discuss these with your doctor if you're taking them or have taken them in the past.

## Antidepressants

According to the *Harvard Review of Psychiatry*, 3.5 percent to 10 percent of women of reproductive age take an antidepressant. Although selective serotonin reuptake inhibitors (SSRIs) are the most commonly prescribed class of antidepressants in pregnancy, these medications do cross the fetal blood-brain barrier, and concerns have been published for years about their safety to developing babies. Animal studies indicate that prenatal exposure to SSRIs impairs development of the serotonin-signaling system in the brain, resulting in impaired working memory, increased aggression, decreased sociability, and decreased maternal behavior in adult offspring—traits that parallel features of neuropsychiatric disorders in humans, including depression, anxiety, and schizophrenia. Other studies have found a two-fold increase in the risk of children developing autism spectrum disorders when their mothers took a SSRI during pregnancy. Furthermore, a recent systematic review found that SSRIs taken for depression during pregnancy also increased the risk of preterm birth.

In addition to their influence on the mood-regulating neurotransmitter serotonin, SSRIs have also been found to increase brain levels of a hormone that stimulates the inhibition of communication between the ovaries and the hypothalamus, the body's master hormone-signaling gland. Inhibiting the hypothalamus' signaling system to the ovaries could result in delayed or lack of ovulation, also known as luteal phase defect.

A recently published report in the *Harvard Review of Psychiatry* noted that six out of seven studies that looked at the effects of SSRIs on male fertility showed negative impacts on sperm parameters.

As depression and anxiety should not go untreated, speak with your doctor about treatment options that are right for you. In many cases, psychotherapy is considered as effective for mild to moderate depression as antidepressants. Nutritional and botanical medicine, acupuncture, and exercise are also effective treatment options to discuss with your practitioner.

## NSAIDs

Non-steroidal anti-inflammatory drugs (NSAIDs) include some of the most common over-the-counter and prescription painkillers, such as ibuprofen and naproxen. Women may take these occasionally for menstrual cramps, head-aches, or migraines, or chronically to control their symptoms of painful or inflammatory conditions. NSAIDs influence the body's balance of a class of hormone-like molecules called prostaglandins, which either promote or decrease inflammation—that's why NSAIDs are effective for pain. Meanwhile, the right prostaglandin balance is needed for fertility-specific functions, such as ovulation and implanta-tion in early pregnancy, to be successful. NSAID medications affect the prostaglandin balance throughout the entire body by way of the bloodstream. This includes the reproductive system, even if that's not the system intended for treatment.

For example, in a cohort study of women with rheumatoid arthritis in Holland, it was found that preconception use of NSAIDs was independently associated with a longer time to achieve pregnancy. In women with juvenile arthritis, taking a daily dose of 500 mg of naproxen has also been shown to impair follicle maturation.

Although ibuprofen is contraindicated after 24 weeks of pregnancy, research suggests possible concerns with first trimester use as well. A 2018 study published in the journal *Human Reproduction* describes that, when fetal ovary sam-ples were exposed to ibuprofen in vitro, it caused cell death and a reduced number of fetal "germ" cells (a female baby's future oocytes).

I realize there's a lot of technical information here, but the underlying message is hopefully clear: If you have pain, it's important to both treat the root cause of the pain and get relief, as well as to understand how any treatments may impact your fertility and pregnancy. Let your practitioner know you're planning to get pregnant, and discuss treatment options that would be appropriate for you, including therapies that could lessen the need for medications, such as an anti-inflammatory diet, acupuncture, physiotherapy, chiropractic care, or osteopathy.

## Metformin

Metformin is commonly prescribed to women with polycystic ovary syndrome (PCOS) in order to restore ovulation. However, it has been found that metformin has weak embryotoxic properties—not what we're looking for! In an IVF study published in the *Journal of Endocrinological Investigation*, women receiving metformin had fewer oocytes retrieved and fertilized and fewer embryos transferred than those who took only oral contraceptives or placebo. The creators of the study concluded that metformin has no positive benefit in IVF for women with PCOS.

However, for women with PCOS, insulin resistance, and hormonal imbalances, metabolic support is needed. A good therapeutic alternative is myo-inositol. In a large open trial conducted in Munich, Germany, in 2018, 3,600 infertile women with PCOS took a supplement of 4000 mg myo-inositol and 400 mcg folic acid daily for an average of 10.2 weeks. After the trial, 70 percent of the women had restored ovulation, and 15 percent of them conceived. Myo-inositol and folic acid supplementation also resulted in beneficial reductions in testosterone and increases in progesterone levels.

In the same trial involving infertile women with PCOS, the researchers then provided the same combination of myo-inositol and folic acid supplements to a sub-group of 14 women with PCOS and compared the effects on the number of oocytes retrieved and fertilized during IVF to those from 15 women with PCOS who were given a placebo. Though more eggs were retrieved in the placebo group, only 43 percent were fertilized; in the inositol group, the ratio of follicles to retrieved oocytes was better, the number of high-grade oocytes was higher, and of the eggs retrieved, 58 percent were fertilized. There were no side effects of inositol and folic acid supplementation. The authors of the trial suggested that myo-inositol is equal to, or more effective than, metformin as an insulin sensitizer in women with PCOS; that it improves egg and embryo quality; and that it may decrease the risk of hyperstimulation syndrome in IVF.

Supplementation with myo-inositol may also have extended benefits through pregnancy in the prevention of gestational diabetes. In a recent clinical trial published in the *European Review for Medical and Pharmacological Sciences*, 68 women took a daily supplement of either 1.75 g myo-inositol, 250 mg D-chiro-inositol, 400 mcg methylated folate (5-MTHF), and other antioxidants or a control treatment of only 400 mcg folic acid from preconception through the 24th week of pregnancy. The women in the inositol group had significantly improved body composition (as measured by body mass index, or BMI) and reduced insulin resistance, compared to the control group.

## Oral Contraceptives

Although it seems counterintuitive, since you may have taken "the pill" or used another form of hormonal birth control for years to *prevent* pregnancy, oral contraceptives are actually a common prescription for short-term use in preparation for IVF. However, studies have found that oral contraceptives deplete important nutrients from the body, like folic acid (folate) and vitamin $B_6$, which are crucial to fertility and pregnancy health—so if you are taking a birth control pill during preconception, it's important to simultaneously replace any potentially depleted nutrients. A good-quality prenatal multivitamin with the active forms of folate and B vitamins, in addition to your fertility-friendly diet, will do the trick.

Don't take the herbal medicine St. John's wort while taking oral contraceptives, as it may increase the speed at which the birth control pill and other hormones are cleared from your body.

## Supplements: The Good, the Bad, and the Useless

In most countries, there aren't tight regulations on what ads can legally claim in terms of the safety and efficacy of natural health products, which, sadly, makes shopping for fertility supplements (retail or online) a bit of a free-for-all. Keep in mind that just because a product is "natural" doesn't mean it's safe or effective for your unique situation. The best evidence that a supplement works comes from clinical trials that involve large enough numbers of participants to obtain meaningful results. In my practice, I recommend to all my patients that we first complete a comprehensive fertility assessment, and then identify the best courses of action, including supplements.

### Dr. Google Is Out

Let's face it: Dr. Google doesn't hear your history, has zero bedside manner, and ends every visit with, "Also, it could be cancer." You deserve to feel heard, supported, and empowered on your path to pregnancy—not led astray by unreliable commentary. Focus on qualified sites where the information is validated. You'll find some good, vetted sites for fertility information in the resources section on page 161. A scientifically sound site won't make you feel anxious or panicky about your situation, nor will it try to sell you something.

## Why Some Supplements Are Particularly Important for Women Undergoing IVF

Following are some supplements that current research shows may be valuable in supporting female fertility, and foods to focus on to obtain these nutrients in the diet, when possible. Remember to discuss any supplements you choose to take with your naturopathic doctor and fertility specialist.

### Iron

Iron is important for follicle growth. UK researchers documented that the more mature follicles closest to ovulation have the ability to take in even more iron in these later stages of development. The Nurses' Health Study showed that women who took iron supplements of 40 mg to 80 mg daily were 40 percent less likely to have infertility than those who didn't take iron. Higher dietary intakes of iron from plant sources, such as beans, nuts, vegetables and fruits—but not meats—were also associated with a lower infertility rate.

As with any supplement, more is not necessarily better. Iron overload causes cell damage, and even small doses of conventional iron supplements can result in stomach upset and constipation, causing many women to abandon them altogether. To make this pill easier to swallow, look for an easier-to-absorb form of this important mineral, such as iron bisglycinate or iron polysaccharide.

## Folic Acid (or Folate)

Folic acid supplementation is encouraged before conception because it significantly decreases the risk of babies being born with neural tube defects (NTDs), such as spina bifida. Also called vitamin $B_9$, folate is used in DNA synthesis and cell division, two processes that happen rapidly from the last stage of egg development through fertilization and early pregnancy. National health authorities encourage women with a low risk of NTD-affected pregnancy to eat a folate-rich diet and to also take a supplement providing 400 mcg folic acid daily for a few months before getting pregnant. According to one obstetrical society, you're considered "low risk" if you've never had a pregnancy where the baby had NTD, and if neither you nor your future baby's father have a personal or family history of NTD. (If you're at high risk for NTD, your doctor will prescribe a daily dose of 1,000 mcg to 4,000 mcg folic acid from preconception to early pregnancy.)

Most "prenatal" supplements provide 1000 mcg folic acid in the daily dose, which actually exceeds the dose that health authorities recognize as safe and effective. Recently, a New York University research report confirmed that there's no additional benefit to low-risk women of taking more than 400 mcg to 800 mcg of folic acid daily.

Due to common and normal genetic variations, up to 60 percent of people cannot convert folic acid (which is synthetic) into the active forms that the body uses. Supplementing with an active form of this vitamin, called methyltetrahydrofolate (L-MTHF), is found to be effective at raising blood folate levels, and since practical ways to screen for the aforementioned gene variations are lacking, choosing to supplement with L-MTHF may be the ideal way to take in adequate levels of folate.

Natural sources of active folate include green vegetables, sprouts, liver, meats, avocados, berries, and brewer's yeast. The U.S. Department of Agriculture estimates that you'll get about 400 mcg folate per 100-gram serving of chicken, lentils, or chickpeas and between 100 mcg and 200 mcg folate from a similar portion of leafy greens, nuts, seeds, quinoa, or eggs.

## Coenzyme Q10

Coenzyme Q10 (CoQ10) is an antioxidant required by the energy-production machinery (called the mitochondria) in eggs to support their ability to grow, avoid chromosomal abnormalities, and build healthy embryos. Eggs contain the highest number of mitochondria of all cell types, but if they can't support these important processes with enough energy, egg quality and the chances of successful pregnancy decrease.

A 2012 study published in *Archives of Gynecology and Obstetrics* showed that CoQ10 is found in follicular fluid, and that women with higher follicular CoQ10 levels had healthier eggs and embryos. Similar findings were reported in a 2017 study in the *Journal of Assisted Reproduction and Genetics*: Among 60 women with unexplained infertility going through IVF, higher follicular CoQ10 levels were found in top-quality embryos, and women who became pregnant had 37 percent higher follicular CoQ10 levels than those who didn't conceive.

In another study published in 2018, a cohort of 15 women aged 31 to 46 years, who experienced infertility for two to four years, took 100 mg CoQ10 twice daily during the month before their next IVF. At retrieval, they had 280 percent higher follicular fluid CoQ10 levels than a similar cohort who didn't supplement with CoQ10.

Foods richest in CoQ10 include organ meats—think skewers of grilled chicken hearts at a traditional Brazilian barbecue. That said, most North Americans don't get much CoQ10 through foods alone. A nutritional survey of 211 men attending the Massachusetts General Hospital Fertility Center for subfertility found that the participant's diets contained an average of about 20 mg CoQ10 daily without supplements. Supplements used in fertility studies range from 200 mg to 800 mg CoQ10 per day, often in divided doses. Some experts recommend checking with your doctor before taking more than 300 mg CoQ10 daily. Rarely, CoQ10 can cause a mild decrease in blood pressure.

## Inositol

Inositols are a group of nutrients that help regulate egg development and optimize the ovarian response to hormonal stimulation. Inositol supplementation has been recommended to increase egg quality in women with PCOS, as well as women going through IVF. One scientific analysis reviewed seven clinical trials involving a total of more than 900 women, and showed that taking inositol supplements in the three months prior to IVF increased the chances of pregnancy by 21 percent.

In *8 Steps to Reverse Your PCOS*, Dr. Fiona McCulloch suggests that the ideal supplement dose would provide the same ratio of inositols as found in the body—that's a ratio of 40:1 myo-inositol to D-chiro-inositol. Following the dosage used in most studies, that would be 4 grams myo-inositol and 100 mg D-chiro-inositol daily, in divided doses.

Out of the nearly 500 foods that have been tested by scientists, fruits, beans, grains, and nuts have been found to contain the highest amounts of myo-inositol. Fresh vegetables and fruits have been found to contain more myo-inositol than frozen or canned versions.

## Vitamin D

Vitamin D is a hormone that's active in the female reproductive system and in fetal programming for the baby's future health. A study of 368 women going through IVF found that vitamin D deficiency was associated with 61 percent lower odds of becoming pregnant. In another study, women with the highest levels of vitamin D had the lowest odds of having preterm birth and low birth weight babies.

Vitamin D is found naturally in cold water fish, and your body naturally produces some vitamin D when your skin is exposed to sunlight. However, vitamin D deficiency is so common that health authorities have called it a pandemic. I recommend a blood test to my patients who are preparing for IVF or trying to conceive, to identify the right dosage of vitamin D needed to reach and maintain a blood level between 100 nmol/L and 150 nmol/L. (The test is called "25-hydroxy D"). If your blood reaches a level above 150 nmol/L, there is a risk for vitamin D overload.

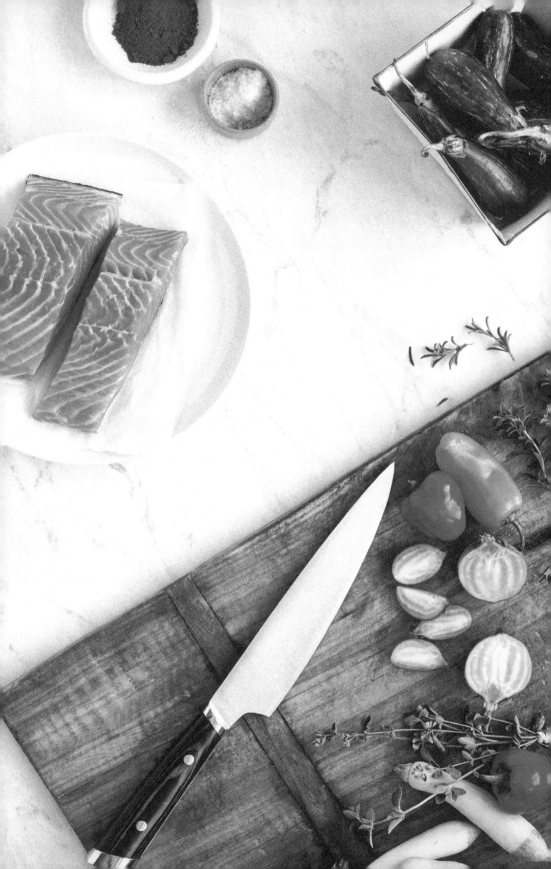

# PART TWO

# The Meal Plans

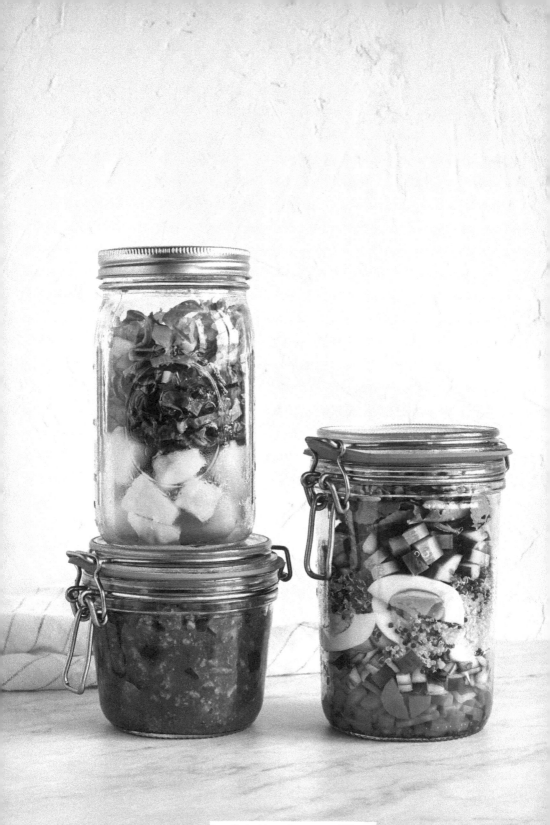

Salad in a Jar, page 90

# CHAPTER THREE

# How to Use the Plans and Recipes

Are you excited? It's time to dive into the meal plans and start enjoying all the nutritional benefits that we've talked about up to this point!

You've learned a tremendous amount about increasing your fertility and your chances for IVF success. Even though there's a lot of information to absorb, we want to set you up for success in your busy, fertility-friendly lifestyle, so Chef Charleston and I have set up your meal plan to be easy as pie. (Speaking of pie, we hope this plan helps you discover some new fertility-friendly comfort foods, too!)

# The Basic Tenets of Eating for Egg Health

Feel free to use the 28-day meal plan just as we've laid it out, or get flexible by mixing and matching based on what's local and in season, which recipes you like the most (whether in this book or not, as long as all ingredients fit with the basic tenets of eating for egg health). Read on to learn more.

## Slow Down Digestion

During the preconception period and into pregnancy, it's important to slow down the rate at which you are stimulating insulin. Slowly digestible carbs will give you slower rises in blood sugar, which means a lower risk of insulin spikes and blood sugar crashes. For a healthy insulin–blood sugar balance, choose whole-grain breads and pastas over white flour products, and enjoy beans, legumes, or root vegetables as sides instead of milled or processed grains like white rice or noodles.

## Eat More Mediterranean

Studies have shown that the Mediterranean diet can increase a couple's chances of IVF pregnancy by up to 40 percent. The catch here is that in these studies, *both* the women and men were eating Mediterranean-style prior to IVF. Compared to other "healthy diets," the Mediterranean diet is lower in red meat and higher in fish, seafood, and poultry; lower in grains and higher in beans and legumes; low in vegetable oils and high in olive oil; and low in processed foods. It also favors fruit for dessert.

The Mediterranean diet features lots of vegetables. Green vegetables are some of the highest sources of folate and calcium. Fill half your plate with low-starch vegetables, such as leafy greens, tomatoes, carrots, green beans, asparagus, mushrooms, sprouts, peppers, onions, garlic, eggplant, or cucumbers. Throughout the week, vary your diet to reflect a full-spectrum rainbow of brightly colored vegetables, from purple eggplants to yellow squash to red bell peppers, as each variety contains a diverse range of nutrients.

Starchy vegetable servings should be about the size of a loose fist. These nutrient-rich sources of carbohydrates include squash, sweet potato, parsnips, potatoes, and beets. You should generally limit grain-based carbs (pasta, bread, crackers, corn, and rice) to portions the size of a tight fist. Loosen that fist a little for a serving size of quinoa (which is actually a seed, not a grain).

## Toss Trans Fats

In the words of my university nutrition professor, trans fats are "potently dangerous molecules." The Nurses' Health Study found that women whose diets contained the highest amounts of trans fats had a greater risk of infertility, compared to the women who consumed the lowest amounts of trans fats. While trace amounts of trans fats are naturally found in dairy products, which are considered beneficial during preconception and IVF, steer clear of hydrogenated or partially hydrogenated vegetable oils, shortening (including in pastries), deep-fried and processed foods, and any other foods that contain trans fats.

## Up the Protein

In a 2009 review, Harvard researchers reinforced the importance of the source of protein for successful fertility. Although
red meat is an excellent source of protein, higher red meat
intake is associated with increased risk of infertility and
lower embryo quality. Instead, the researchers suggest, pri-
oritize poultry, low-toxin fish and seafood, and vegetarian
sources of protein, including free-range eggs, organic soy,
legumes, beans, nuts, and seeds. Choose low-mercury fish
such as wild-caught Alaskan or sockeye salmon, anchovies,
sardines, shrimp, crab, mussels, line-caught albacore tuna,
Atlantic mackerel, and pollock. Avoid high-mercury fish like
shark, swordfish, tuna (other than albacore), king mackerel,
marlin, and grouper. See the resources section (page 161) for
information about fish and seafood choices that are safer for
preconception and pregnancy.

## Use Fertility-Friendly Fats

Many types of fats (with the exception of trans fats and the
list of oils to avoid on page 16) are actually good for us. Fats
slow the rate of carbohydrates absorbing into the bloodstream, keep us feeling fuller longer, make our food taste more
delicious and satisfying, and provide a source of energy that
doesn't raise insulin. The Nurses' Health Study shows us that
women who include dairy products in their diets have a lower
risk of ovulatory infertility when they have higher intakes of
full-fat dairy as opposed to skim or low-fat versions. Important

nutrients like CoQ10 and vitamins A, E, D, and K$_2$ are best absorbed when dietary fats are present. And every type of cell, including eggs, needs good-quality fats—including saturated fats and omega-3s—to plug into its membrane to protect the DNA inside and ensure optimal function. Extra-virgin olive oil is a mainstay in this book's IVF-friendly meal plans. Omega-3 oils from fish and fish oil supplements help to create a less inflammatory environment in the body, and higher intakes of these oils are associated with a lower risk of infertility. A serving of healthy fat equals 1 to 2 tablespoons extra-virgin olive oil, half an avocado, a tablespoon of organic butter or ghee, 2 tablespoons nut or seed butter, ¼ cup nuts or seeds, or a piece of organic cheese the size of your thumb.

## Hydrate Wisely

At least half of my patients tell me they *know* they need to drink more water. But did you know that any caffeinated beverage counts as a "minus one" glass of water against your day's quota? Data clearly shows that sweetened beverages like pop or soda are among the most anti-fertility foods women can consume. This may be because sugary beverages cause spikes in insulin, and perhaps because drinking them displaces the water your body needs for everything to function properly. If you can relate, now's the time to make new habits! Drink 8 to 10 glasses of filtered water daily—spruce it up with a wedge of lemon, a few frozen berries, or a sprig of fresh mint (spearmint is a good choice, especially for women with PCOS).

# THE IVF DIET FOOD PYRAMID

A successful daily and weekly fertility-friendly meal plan looks like this:

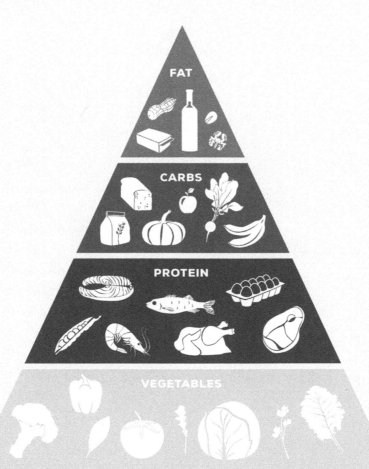

**FAT**
Olive Oil, Butter and Ghee, Coconut Oil, Nuts and Seeds, Nut and Seed Butters

**CARB**
Whole Grains, Root Vegetables, Fruit

**PROTEIN**
Fish and Seafood, Legumes, Eggs, Protein Powder and Meats, Including Liver and Other Organ Meats

**VEGETABLES**
Green and Colorful Vegetables

## Tips and Recommendations for Getting Through the Meal Plan

Any change—even a positive one; even one you ENJOY—can feel hard just because it's different, as our brain naturally resists anything out of the norm. I always suggest to clients that they follow the 80/20 rule. If you follow this plan 80 percent of the time, you will still get results! Let's not label the other 20 percent as "cheating." If you decide to eat a non-IVF-friendly food during that other 20 percent of the time, please sit down, be present, and allow yourself to truly enjoy it. Then simply return to the plan at your next meal or snack. Feeling guilty and labeling a single indulgent choice as "cheating" has actually been shown to disrupt hormones and drive cravings.

Keep in mind any individual factors that may require you to revise this plan. In the recipes, we've identified easy ways to substitute certain ingredients or to work around food allergies or sensitivities. If you're not sure what foods you're sensitive to, consult a naturopathic doctor and look into a food intolerance test, which screens for inappropriately high levels of antibodies your immune system is creating in response to certain foods.

## Tips for Eating Out

My husband jokes that he'd never go on *The Amazing Race* with me, because we'd be so unfocused at pit stops with all my food questions ("Can I get that gluten-free?" "Is the fish local?" "Do you have unsweetened almond milk?") that we'd be lost before even starting. Well, the joke's on him, because not only would I crush it on that show, but, also, restaurants are simply way more substitution-savvy than ever before. It's no longer a big deal to ask your server to make your order:

- ▼ unsweetened
- ▼ caffeine-free
- ▼ bunless or breadless
- ▼ grilled instead of fried
- ▼ gluten-free
- ▼ dairy-free
- ▼ ... etc., to get it just right for you and your specific needs.

As you wrap your head around your new food goals, consider expanding your culinary horizons when dining out. Some of my favorite go-to restaurant dishes include:

**Mediterranean**—kebabs, hummus, grilled vegetables, souvlaki

**Thai**—red, yellow, or green curry with vegetables and a protein; pad Thai; spicy soups

**Japanese**—sushi, soups, veggie and fish dishes

**Indian**—spicy curry, lentils, papadum, tandoori

**Vegetarian**—soups, salads, wraps, stir-fry with a protein

**Soups**—the more homemade, the better

**Barbecue**—grilled meat or fish with vegetables and a baked potato

# SHOPPING LIST USER GUIDE

The shopping list we provide with each weekly meal plan will give you everything you'll need to create a full week's worth of meals. We've organized the shopping lists using the sections of any typical grocery store, so you can easily map out your trip (or save even more time and simply point and click to order everything online from your favorite grocery delivery service).

Clients often ask me how important it is to go organic. I've included the Environmental Working Group's Dirty Dozen™ and Clean Fifteen™ lists, which indicate, respectively, the fruits and vegetables that contain the highest concentrations of pesticides and those that are least likely to be contaminated (see page 159). If your budget allows, I recommend sourcing animal foods from free-range or organic farms where the animals are raised on the healthiest diets, such as grass (not grain) for cows and insects and worms (in addition to grains and seeds) for hens. Pasture-raised and organic animal foods are likely to be higher in beneficial nutrients and lower in harmful residues like antibiotics, hormones, and pesticides. If organic or grass-fed meat isn't an option for you, choose the leanest cuts and remove visible fat before cooking, as toxins tend to be stored in the animals' fat.

For perishables such as fresh produce and meat and fish, my husband and I like to snap up local, organic, or pasture-raised foods whenever they're on sale and freeze them until we're ready to cook them. If you do this, you'll want to plan ahead for when you'll thaw your frozen foods before you cook.

# Week 1 Meal Plan

Note: If you have dietary restrictions, just follow the plan as written and use the substitution notes found in the individual recipes to fit your needs.

## Shopping List

### Pantry

- Anchovies, 1 can
- Basil, dried
- Bay leaves
- Black pepper
- Bread, whole-grain or gluten-free, 1 loaf
- Brown rice, quinoa or millet
- Cacao nibs
- Cacao powder, raw
- Capers, ¼ cup
- Cayenne pepper
- Chia seeds, ½ cup
- Chicken or vegetable stock, 3¼ quarts
- Chili powder
- Coconut, unsweet-ened shredded
- Coconut oil, 1 jar

- Collagen or gelatin powder, 1 package
- Coriander seed, ground
- Corn tortillas, 1 package
- Crackers, whole-grain, 1 box
- Croutons, 1 package (optional)
- Cumin, ground
- Garlic, 2 heads
- Garlic powder
- Ginger, ground
- Honey
- Maple syrup, pure
- Mayonnaise, avocado oil, 2 cups
- Mint, dried
- Mustard, Dijon

- Nut butter (almond, cashew, peanut—your choice)
- Oats, gluten-free rolled
- Olive oil, extra virgin
- Onions, red (2)
- Onions, white (2)
- Oregano, dried
- Paprika
- Protein powder, vanilla
- Red pepper flakes
- Red wine vinaigrette
- Roasted red peppers, 1 jar

- Sea salt (fine)
- Seeds and nuts, ½ cup
- Quinoa
- Tomatoes, crushed, 1 (14-ounce) can
- Tomatoes, diced, 3 (14-ounce) cans
- Thyme, dried
- Turmeric, ground
- Vanilla extract, pure
- Vinegar, balsamic
- Vinegar, apple cider
- Walnuts

## Refrigerator and Freezer

- Almond milk, unsweetened, 1 quart
- Apple, 1
- Avocados, 6
- Bananas, 2
- Basil
- Bell peppers, any color, 4
- Bell peppers, red, 2
- Cod fillets, black, 3
- Blueberries, 1 pint

- Bones, 4 (such as chicken, turkey, or beef)
- Carrots, 1 pound
- Celery, 1 bunch
- Cheese, goat, 1 log
- Chicken or lamb, 1¼ pounds
- Chicken thighs, bone-in, 8
- Cilantro

- Coconut water, 2 quarts
- Cream, heavy (whipping), 1 pint, or full-fat coconut milk, 4 (14-ounce) cans
- Cucumbers, 3
- Dill, fresh
- Eggs, pasture-raised, 2 dozen
- Ghee or clarified butter
- Ginger
- Kale, 2 bunches
- Leek, 1
- Lemon juice, ¼ cup
- Lemons, 6
- Lettuce, romaine, 4 heads
- Limes, 5
- Mango, frozen, 1 pound
- Mozzarella, buffalo, 1 ball
- Mushrooms, cremini, 1 cup
- Mushrooms, oyster, 1 cup
- Mushrooms, shiitake, 1 cup
- Pineapple, fresh or frozen, 2 cups
- Salad greens, fresh, (e.g., baby kale, spinach, romaine lettuce, etc.)
- Spinach, baby, or baby kale, 4 cups
- Strawberries, fresh, 1 pint
- Strawberries, frozen, 1 pound
- Sun-dried tomatoes, 1 jar
- Tomatoes, 2
- Turkey, ground, 3 pounds
- Yogurt, Greek, unsweetened, or coconut yogurt, unsweetened, 4 cups
- Zucchini, 3

# DAY 1

BREAKFAST: Chocolate Monkey Smoothie (page 82)

LUNCH: Salad in a Jar (page 90), piece of fruit

DINNER: Mediterranean Kebabs (page 116)

TIME-SAVING TIP: Prep Overnight Oats with Fresh Fruit (page 84) and Chia Chocolate Pudding (page 129) for the next day.

# DAY 2

BREAKFAST: Overnight Oats with Fresh Fruit (page 84)

LUNCH: Leftovers from Mediterranean Kebabs, piece of fruit

DINNER: Cream of Mushroom Soup (page 93), Caprese Salad (page 92), Chia Chocolate Pudding (page 129)

TIME-SAVING TIP: Chop vegetables for tomorrow's dinner Barbecue Chicken with Veggie Kebabs, (page 113).

# DAY 3

BREAKFAST: Avocado Toast (page 86)

LUNCH: Leftovers from Cream of Mushroom Soup, whole-grain crackers

DINNER: Barbecue Chicken with Veggie Kebabs (page 113)

TIME-SAVING TIP: Reserve the chicken bones from dinner. Make Caesar Dressing (page 135) and prep chicken Caesar in a jar. (Put the dressing in the jar first, followed by leftover chilled barbecue chicken, then fresh greens.)

# DAY 4

BREAKFAST: Tropical Green Smoothie (page 83)
LUNCH: Prepared Chicken Caesar in a jar, piece of crusty bread
DINNER: Beanless Turkey Chili (page 103), Strawberry-Mango Compote (page 126)
TIME-SAVING TIP: Make Basic Bone Broth (page 120) using the leftover bones from Barbecue Chicken.

# DAY 5

BREAKFAST: Strawberry-Mango Compote (page 126) with yogurt, cup of Basic Bone Broth (page 120)
LUNCH: Leftovers from Beanless Turkey Chili
DINNER: Chicken Cacciatore with Kale Caesar Salad (page 110), noodles (if desired)
TIME-SAVING TIP: Hard-boil eggs for snacks and chop carrot and celery sticks.

# DAY 6

BREAKFAST: Chocolate Monkey Smoothie (page 82)
LUNCH: Leftovers from Chicken Cacciatore
DINNER: Blackened Fish Tacos (page 99), Zesty Guacamole (page 136)
TIME-SAVING TIP: Chop vegetables for tomorrow's Zucchini and Roasted Red Pepper Omelet.

# DAY 7

BREAKFAST: Tropical Green Smoothie (page 83)

LUNCH: Taco Chips (page 130) and Zesty Guacamole (page 136), cup of Basic Bone Broth (page 120), piece of fruit

DINNER: Zucchini and Roasted Red Pepper Omelet (page 95), Avocado Toast (page 86)

TIME-SAVING TIP: Prep Overnight Oats with Fresh Fruit (page 84), Veggie Western Sandwich (page 96), and Salad in a Jar (page 90).

# SUGGESTED SNACKS

Veggie sticks and Zesty Guacamole (page 136)

Nuts and berries

Celery sticks and nut butter

Chia Chocolate Pudding (page 129)

Hard-boiled eggs and carrot sticks

# Week 2 Meal Plan

Note: If you have dietary restrictions, just follow the plan as written and use the substitution notes found in the individual recipes to fit your needs.

## Shopping List

### Pantry

- Almonds, 2 cups
- Almonds, sliced, ¼ cup
- Blueberries, dried, ½ cup
- Bread, whole-grain or gluten-free, 2 loaves
- Capers
- Chia seeds, 1 cup
- Chicken stock, 3 liters
- Chickpeas, 2 (15-ounce) cans
- Cinnamon, ground
- Coconut, unsweetened shredded
- Cumin, ground
- Curry powder
- Dates, Medjool, 1 package

- Flaxseed, 1 tablespoon
- Garlic, 1 head
- Oats, gluten-free rolled, ½ cup
- Oil, coconut
- Onions, white, 3
- Paprika
- Pecans, 2 cups
- Pecans, chopped, ¼ cup
- Pumpkin seeds, ½ cup
- Red curry paste, Thai, 1 jar
- Red pepper flakes
- Roasted red peppers, 1 jar
- Sea salt (fine)

- Seeds and nuts, ½ cup
- Sesame oil, 1 teaspoon
- Sesame seeds, ¼ cup for garnish
- Shallots, 5
- Sunflower seeds, ½ cup
- Tahini
- Tamari
- Vinegar, apple cider
- Walnuts, 2 cups

## Refrigerator and Freezer

- Cucumbers, 2
- Dill, 1 bunch
- Frozen blueberries, 1½ pounds
- Frozen mango, 1 pound
- Frozen or fresh pineapple, 2 cups
- Frozen diced pre-cooked squash, 1 cup
- Frozen strawberries, 2 pounds
- Ginger, 2 pieces
- Goat cheese, 8 tablespoons
- Grapes, 1 bunch
- Ground turkey, 1 pound
- Kale, 3 bunches
- Leek, 1

# DAY 1

**BREAKFAST:** Overnight Oats with Fresh Fruit (page 84)

**LUNCH:** Veggie Western Sandwich (page 96), Salad in a Jar (page 90)

**DINNER:** Coconut Curry Chicken (page 106), Green Salad (page 91), Basil-Berry Swirl Sorbet (page 128)

**TIME-SAVING TIP:** Make Seedy Granola (page 122) and chop carrots and celery sticks for snacks throughout the week.

## DAY 2

BREAKFAST: Chia Chocolate Pudding (page 129)
LUNCH: Leftovers from Coconut Curry Chicken
DINNER: Slow Cooker Pulled Chicken (page 108), coleslaw
TIME-SAVING TIP: Prep Salad in a Jar (page 90): Put the
dressing into the jar first, followed by the leftover pulled
chicken and fresh greens. Make Creamy Hummus (page 137).

## DAY 3

BREAKFAST: Tropical Green Smoothie (page 83)
LUNCH: Leftovers from Slow Cooker Pulled Chicken, Salad
in a Jar (page 90)
DINNER: Dill Baked Salmon (page 102), Green Salad (page 91)
TIME-SAVING TIP: Prep Salad in a Jar (page 90) using
leftover Dill Baked Salmon.

## DAY 4

BREAKFAST: Chocolate Monkey Smoothie (page 82)
LUNCH: Salad in a Jar (page 90) with leftover Dill
Baked Salmon
DINNER: Cream of Mushroom Soup (page 93), Caprese
Salad (page 92), piece of crusty bread, Strawberry-Mango
Compote (page 126)
TIME-SAVING TIP: Make Maple Toasted Trail Mix (page 124),
chop veggie sticks.

# DAY 5

BREAKFAST: Strawberry-Mango Compote (page 126), nuts, yogurt

LUNCH: Leftovers from Cream of Mushroom Soup, veggie sticks, piece of fruit

DINNER: Zucchini and Roasted Red Pepper Omelet (page 95), Avocado Toast (page 86)

TIME-SAVING TIP: Prep Veggie Western Sandwich (page 96).

# DAY 6

BREAKFAST: Tropical Green Smoothie (page 83)

LUNCH: Veggie Western Sandwich (page 96), veggie sticks

DINNER: Turkey Meatballs (page 104), Fresh Berries and Cream (page 127)

TIME-SAVING TIP: Chop veggies for Scallop and Broccoli Stir-Fry (page 97).

# DAY 7

BREAKFAST: Maple Toasted Trail Mix (page 124), yogurt

LUNCH: Turkey Meatball Sandwich (page 105)

DINNER: Scallop and Broccoli Stir-Fry (page 97), Basil-Berry Swirl Sorbet (page 128)

TIME-SAVING TIP: Prep Beanless Turkey Chili (page 103) for the slow cooker, chop veggie sticks.

# SUGGESTED SNACKS

Apples and cheese

Seedy Granola (page 122)

Celery sticks and nut butter

Veggie sticks and Creamy Hummus (page 137)

Chia Chocolate Pudding (page 129)

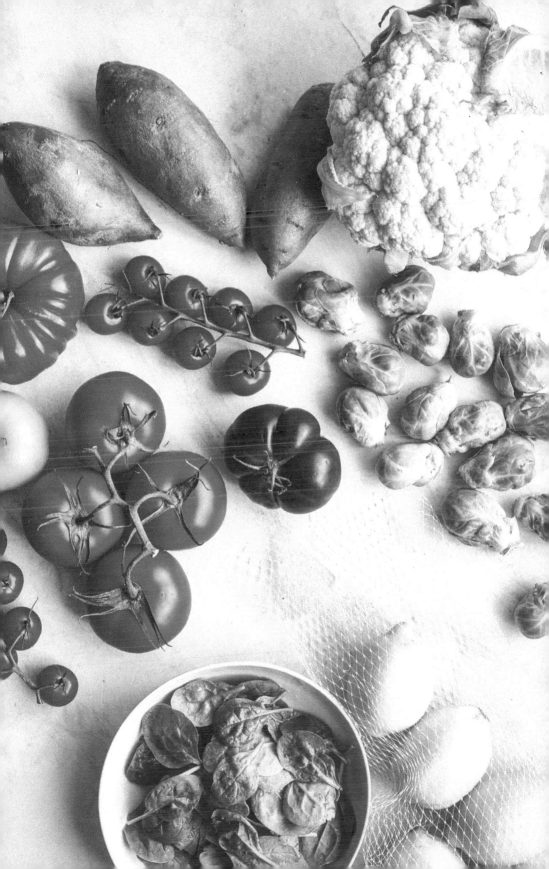

# Week 3 Meal Plan

Note: If you have dietary restrictions, just follow the plan as written and use the substitution notes found in the individual recipes to fit your needs.

## Shopping List

### Pantry

- Almonds, 2 cups
- Blueberries, dried, ½ cup
- Bread, whole-grain or gluten-free, 2 loaves
- Cacao nibs
- Chicken or vegetable stock, 2 liters
- Coconut, unsweetened, shredded, ¾ cup
- Corn tortillas, 1 package
- Crackers, whole-grain, 1 box
- Dates, Medjool, 1 package
- Garlic, fresh, 2 heads
- Maple syrup, pure
- Onions, white, 5
- Pecans, 2 cups
- Red wine vinaigrette
- Seeds and nuts, ¼ cup
- Thyme, dried
- Tomatoes, crushed, 1 (14-ounce) can
- Tomatoes, diced, 3 (14-ounce) cans
- Walnuts, 2 cups

## Refrigerator and Freezer

- Almond milk, unsweetened, 1 quart
- Apple, 1
- Avocados, 3
- Bananas, 2
- Basil, 2 bunches
- Bell peppers, red, 2
- Blackberries, 1 pint
- Blueberries, 1 pint
- Blueberries, frozen, 1 pound
- Carrots, 5
- Celery, 2 bunches
- Chicken thighs, boneless and skinless, 6 pounds
- Coconut milk, 2 quarts
- Coconut milk, unsweetened, 1 quart
- Coconut water, 1 quart
- Cod fillets, black, 3
- Cream, heavy (whipping), 1 cup
- Cucumber, 1
- Dill

- Eggs, pasture-raised, 2 dozen
- Ginger, 2 pieces
- Grapes, 1 pint
- Kale, 1 bunch
- Leek, 1
- Lemons, 2
- Lettuce, romaine, 2 heads
- Limes, 4
- Mango, frozen, 1 pound
- Mint
- Mushrooms, cremini, 1 cup
- Mushrooms, oyster, 1 cup
- Mushrooms, shiitake, 1 cup
- Orange juice
- Pineapple, fresh or frozen, 2 cups
- Raspberries, 1 pint
- Salad greens
- Salmon, Pacific or sockeye, 4 fillets
- Spinach, baby, or baby kale

- Strawberries, frozen,
  1½ pounds
- Turkey, ground,
  3 pounds

- Yogurt, Greek,
  unsweetened, or
  coconut milk yogurt,
  unsweetened, 2 quarts
- Zucchini, 2

# DAY 1

**BREAKFAST:** Tropical Green Smoothie (page 83)

**LUNCH:** Leftovers from Scallop and Broccoli Stir-Fry

**DINNER:** Beanless Turkey Chili (page 103), Fresh Berries and Cream (page 127)

**TIME-SAVING TIP:** Hard boil eggs, prep eggs with Salad in a Jar (page 90).

# DAY 2

**BREAKFAST:** Maple Toasted Trail Mix (page 124), yogurt

**LUNCH:** Eggs over Salad in a Jar (page 90)

**DINNER:** Mediterranean Kebabs (page 116) and grilled vegetables; Strawberry-Mango Compote (page 126)

**TIME-SAVING TIP:** Chop carrot sticks.

# DAY 3

BREAKFAST: Chocolate Monkey Smoothie (page 82)

LUNCH: Leftovers from Mediterranean Kebabs and grilled vegetables

DINNER: Blackened Fish Tacos (page 99) and Zesty Guacamole (page 136), Berry-Basil Swirl Sorbet (page 128)

TIME-SAVING TIP: Make Basic Bone Broth (page 120), prep Salad in a Jar (page 90), make Taco Chips (page 130).

# DAY 4

BREAKFAST: Avocado Toast (page 86)

LUNCH: Taco Chips (page 130) and Zesty Guacamole (page 136), cup of Basic Bone Broth, Salad in a Jar (page 90)

DINNER: Chicken Cacciatore with noodles, Kale Caesar Salad (page 110)

TIME-SAVING TIP: Chop celery sticks.

# DAY 5

BREAKFAST: Tropical Green Smoothie (page 83)

LUNCH: Leftovers from Chicken Cacciatore and noodles

DINNER: Dill Baked Salmon (page 102), Green Salad (page 91)

TIME-SAVING TIP: Chop veggies for Veggie Western Sandwich (page 96).

## DAY 6

BREAKFAST: Veggie Western Sandwich (page 96)
LUNCH: Leftover Dill Baked Salmon on whole-grain crackers, Salad in a Jar (page 90)
DINNER: Cream of Mushroom Soup (page 93), Kale Caesar Salad (page 110)
TIME-SAVING TIP: Hard-boil eggs.

## DAY 7

BREAKFAST: Maple Toasted Trail Mix (page 124), yogurt
LUNCH: Eggs over Salad in a Jar (page 90)
DINNER: Slow Cooker Pulled Chicken (page 108) and coleslaw, Basil-Berry Swirl Sorbet (page 128)
TIME-SAVING TIP: Put Tropical Green Smoothie (page 83) ingredients in blender jar and refrigerate until ready to blend tomorrow.

## SUGGESTED SNACKS

Maple Toasted Trail Mix (page 124)
Nuts and berries
Hard-boiled egg and carrot sticks
Celery sticks and nut butter

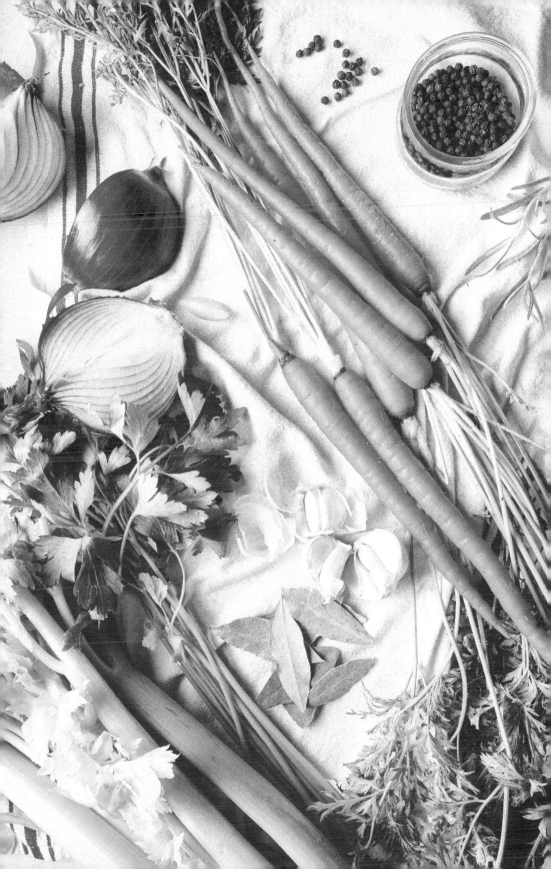

# Week 4 Meal Plan

Note: If you have dietary restrictions, just follow the plan as written and use the substitution notes found in the individual recipes to fit your needs.

## Shopping List

### Pantry

- Almonds, sliced, ½ cup
- Bread, whole-grain or gluten-free, 2 loaves
- Cacao powder
- Capers
- Chia seeds, ½ cup
- Chicken stock
- Chickpeas, 1 (15-ounce) can
- Coconut oil
- Coconut, unsweetened, shredded, 1 cup
- Dates, Medjool, 7
- Flaxseed, 2 tablespoons
- Garlic, fresh, 1 head
- Honey
- Maple syrup, pure
- Oats, gluten-free rolled, 1 cup
- Onions, red, 2
- Onions, white, 3
- Pecans, ½ cup
- Pumpkin seeds, 1 cup
- Red curry paste, Thai, 1 jar
- Roasted red peppers, 1 jar
- Seeds and nuts, ¼ cup
- Shallots, 3
- Sun-dried tomatoes, 1 jar

- Sunflower
seeds, 1 cup
- Tomato paste, 1
(6-ounce) can

- Tomatoes, diced, 1
(28-ounce) can
- Vanilla extract, pure

## Refrigerator and Freezer

- Almond milk,
unsweetened, 2 liters
- Apples, 4
- Asparagus, 1 bunch
- Avocados, 5
- Bananas, 2
- Basil, 1 bunch
- Bell peppers, 2
- Blackberries, 1 pint
- Blueberries, 1 pint
- Blueberries,
frozen, 3 cups
- Broccoli crowns, 2
- Carrots, 10
- Cheese, goat, 1 log
- Cheese, organic,
1 block
- Chicken, bone-
less and skinless,
5 pounds
- Cilantro, 1 bunch

- Coconut milk,
unsweetened, 2 liters
- Coconut water, 1 cup
- Cucumbers, 3
- Dill, 1 bunch
- Eggs, pasture-raised,
3 dozen
- Ghee or clarified
butter, ¼ cup
- Ginger
- Grapes, 1 bunch
- Kale, 2 bunches
- Leek, 1
- Lemons, 4
- Lettuce, romaine,
1 head
- Limes
- Mango, frozen,
1 pound
- Mint
- Mushrooms,
cremini, 1 cup

- Mushrooms, oyster, 1 cup
- Mushrooms, shiitake, 1 cup
- Pineapple, fresh or frozen, 2 cups
- Raspberries, 1 pint
- Salad greens
- Scallops, baby bay, 1 pound
- Spinach, baby or baby kale, 5 cups

- Squash, frozen, diced, and precooked, 1½ cups
- Strawberries, frozen, 1½ pounds
- Turkey, ground, 1 pound
- Yogurt, Greek unsweetened, or coconut milk yogurt, 4 cups
- Zucchini, 2

# DAY 1

**BREAKFAST:** Tropical Green Smoothie (page 83)
**LUNCH:** Leftovers from Pulled Chicken and coleslaw
**DINNER:** Scallop and Broccoli Stir-Fry (page 97), Strawberry-Mango Compote (page 126)
**TIME-SAVING TIP:** Make Chia Chocolate Pudding (page 129).

# DAY 2

**BREAKFAST:** Chia Chocolate Pudding (page 129)
**LUNCH:** Leftovers from Scallop and Broccoli Stir-Fry
**DINNER:** Coconut Curry Chicken (page 106), Green Salad (page 91), piece of fruit
**TIME-SAVING TIPS:** Make Seedy Granola (page 122).

# DAY 3

BREAKFAST: Seedy Granola (page 122)

LUNCH: Leftovers from Coconut Curry Chicken

DINNER: Cream of Mushroom Soup (page 93),
piece of crusty bread

TIME-SAVING TIP: Chop veggies for Barbecue Chicken with
Veggie Kebabs (page 113).

# DAY 4

BREAKFAST: Chocolate Monkey Smoothie (page 82)

LUNCH: Leftovers from Cream of Mushroom Soup

DINNER: Barbecue Chicken with Veggie Kebabs (page 113),
Fresh Berries and Cream (page 127)

TIME-SAVING TIP: Prep Salad in a Jar (page 90) with
leftover cooled barbecue chicken.

# DAY 5

BREAKFAST: Avocado Toast (page 86)

LUNCH: Leftover Barbecue Chicken over Salad in a Jar
(page 90), piece of fruit

DINNER: Chicken Cacciatore with Kale Caesar Salad
(page 110)

TIME-SAVING TIP: Chop veggie sticks.

# DAY 6

BREAKFAST: Leftover Seedy Granola
LUNCH: Leftovers from Chicken Cacciatore
DINNER: Turkey Meatballs (page 104), Basil-Berry Swirl
Sorbet (page 128)
TIME-SAVING TIP: Make Creamy Hummus (page 137),
prep veggies for Zucchini and Roasted Red Pepper
Omelet (page 95).

# DAY 7

BREAKFAST: Chocolate Monkey Smoothie (page 82)
LUNCH: Turkey Meatball Sandwich (page 97)
DINNER: Zucchini and Roasted Red Pepper Omelet
(page 95), Avocado Toast (page 86), Fresh Berries and
Cream (page 127)

# SUGGESTED SNACKS

Hard-boiled egg and carrot sticks
Apples and cheese
Chia Chocolate Pudding (page 129)
Veggie sticks and Creamy Hummus (page 137)
Seedy Granola (page 122)
Veggie sticks and Zesty Guacamole (page 136)

# Adjusting for Medical Considerations

The right diet for you can be as individualized as you are, especially if you have a health condition requiring treatment or nutritional guidelines.

## If You Have Endometriosis

Endometriosis is estimated to affect 25 to 40 percent of infertile women. As a result of a combination of hormonal imbalances, especially excess estrogen activity, and inflammatory and autoimmune factors, this inflammatory condition occurs when endometrial tissue is implanted at sites of the reproductive system other than the lining of the uterus, including the fallopian tubes, ovaries, or the pelvic organs. Researchers have found that women with endometriosis may have lower quantity and quality of eggs and embryos with IVF because of the level of inflammation and molecular stress on their ovaries, oocytes, and DNA. If you have endometriosis, include plenty of cruciferous vegetables (broccoli, cauliflower, kale, and rapini) in your diet, supply your gut with friendly bacteria, such as the probiotic *Lactobacillus rhamnosus*, and eat foods with plenty of soluble fiber and phytoestrogens, like a few teaspoons of ground flaxseed added to your smoothie or oatmeal, to keep hormones in a healthier balance.

## If You Have PCOS

Polycystic ovary syndrome, or PCOS, is the most common female hormone disorder in the world—and it is also a key condition that leads women to require fertility support. As women with PCOS are more prone to insulin resistance and inflammation, if you have this condition, consider reducing your intake of refined sugar, dairy, and red meat. Fertility-friendly diets typically include reduced amounts of these food categories, and you'll find that our meal plans follow this, too, by including poultry-based variations of traditionally red meat dishes, dairy-free options, and no refined sugar.

## If You Have Diabetes or Can't Have Sugar

If you're watching your sugar, this meal plan is ideal for you! If you've been directed by your medical practitioner to follow an ultra-low-carb diet, be sure to follow up with them to obtain specifics for how to replace carbohydrates with fat and protein. Our meal plan is designed to be "adequate" in carbohydrates, which is lower carbohydrate than most "healthy" diets, and certainly lower than the standard American diet. You'll see there is no refined sugar in any of the recipes, and even nutritious sweeteners like honey and maple syrup are optional or used sparingly. Artificial sweeteners have been shown to raise insulin levels (even though they don't contain any sugar) and may even be carcinogenic. You got it—avoid!

## If You Can't Have Dairy

Thankfully, most grocery stores stock plenty of nondairy milks, creams, butters, cheeses, and even yogurts. Here are some easy substitutions to use in the recipes in this book:

▼ Alternative milks for smoothies include almond, coconut, organic soy, hemp, or cashew milks. You can also easily make your own delicious nut milk by blending raw, soaked nuts in water.

▼ Whipped cream can be replaced with whipped coconut cream.

▼ Nutritional yeast can substitute for Parmesan cheese.

## If You've Had Unsuccessful IVF Cycles

You're not alone. Without additional support, IVF on its own can provide a couple about a 30 percent chance of bringing home a baby after an average of four cycles. It's often a necessary medical technology, but IVF was never intended to be the standalone answer to all fertility challenges. Use this book as a starting point to make lifestyle shifts that can help you increase your chances of having a healthy pregnancy and baby. You really can change your physiology in just a few months' time, and your next IVF cycle will be a new opportunity, because you're bringing an even healthier self to the cycle!

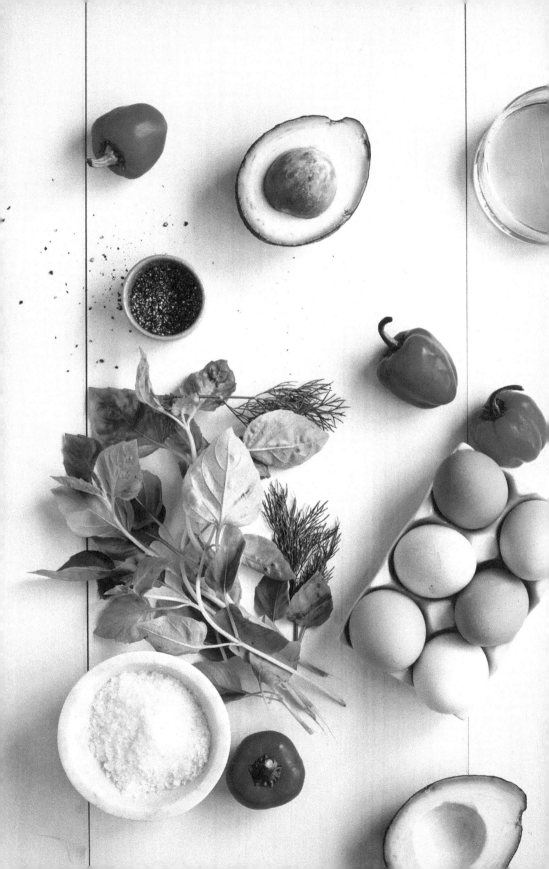

# CHAPTER FOUR

# Recipes for Success

The two most common issues I see in my patients who are struggling with egg quality issues, whether they want to conceive naturally or with assisted reproduction technology, is that otherwise "healthy" diets leave them lacking in micro-nutrients (vitamins, minerals, essential fats, and antioxidants) and with excesses of certain macronutrients (usually carbo-hydrates, such as sugars). Even health-conscious versions of the standard North American diet are leaving women at risk of having eggs that can't quite keep up with the energy demands of maturation, fertilization, and early embryonic cell division. Women's hormones can also shift out of balance, especially if they have high levels of insulin.

Insulin is required to drive glucose and amino acids, which are absorbed from carbohydrate and protein foods, respec-tively, into your cells to allow them to function. If you eat too many carbs and/or protein in a meal or eat too frequently, you risk developing high insulin levels. Eventually, if your insulin levels are too high, your cells grow resistant to insulin's continuous knock-knock-knocking at their doors, and they stop responding to the insulin. Your body continues to pro-duce more insulin, and your cells continue to reject it. When this happens, your body reaches a metabolic state called "insulin resistance," which is a problem for fertility because it's associated with excess inflammation, estrogen production, and weight gain. When insulin is too high, the actions of tes-tosterone increase in the ovary, causing dysfunction in follicle growth and prevention of normal ovulation.

# Breakfast Really Is the Most Important Meal of the Day

A 2013 study showed that the timing and size of meals can have a dramatic effect on hormone balance and follicle development in lean women with PCOS who consumed an 1,800-calorie daily diet. In this study, the women who ate a large breakfast, medium-size lunch, and small dinner had 54 percent healthier insulin levels, 50 percent lower testosterone, 105 percent lower sex-hormone-binding globulin, and an improved ovulation rate compared with those who consumed the same total calories each day with a small breakfast, medium-size lunch, and large dinner.

While most of us may not have an appetite (or even a schedule) that can accommodate a big breakfast daily, I wanted you to know that there is some good science behind the old adage that "breakfast is the most important meal of the day." To help keep insulin (and all the hormones it influences) in check, focus on building your meals and snacks around a protein, add a fertility-friendly fat, and then include a small amount of carbohydrate. Protein stimulates the release of insulin, but together with fat, it adds to the feeling of satisfaction and helps anchor your blood sugar for the day. Protein at breakfast is especially important. You'll need to get 20 to 25 grams of protein with each meal to keep things in a healthy balance. Here are some additional tips:

> **Prevent deprivation.** Eat enough at each meal that you can go four or five hours before you're hungry again. Giving your system a break between meals or snacks allows other hormones to come on board and keep insulin in balance.

**Don't crash.** Getting "hangry" isn't good for anyone! If you know you'll go longer than 5 hours between meals and you're hungry, have a snack. See chapter 7 (page 119) and pages 49, 54, 60, and 66 for snack suggestions that you can use as templates. Anchor your snacks with some protein and fat. If you're exercising, have some complex carbs with your post-workout snack, such as half a banana in a protein shake.

**Sack the sugar.** The Nurses' Health Study showed that refined carbs (including sugar, carbonated soft drinks, and baked goods), are one of the most harmful food categories to female fertility, with the highest intakes being a risk factor for ovulatory infertility. If you're craving something sweet, try one of the treats in chapter 7 (page 119), or enjoy a small serving of fresh fruit with a meal.

## Altering Cell Structure Is Hard Work

Healing is always possible, but think of it as a journey. Your body is miraculous, yet change doesn't usually happen overnight. Your body innately knows how to use the good nutrients you're eating to shift you toward your optimal fertile state. It also knows how to release obstacles like toxins, especially when it's well nourished and less stressed. Watch for what I call "microchanges": Are you typically in a better mood or have a higher energy level by the end of the day? Are you sleeping a little more deeply? Is your period a little easier? Has your libido or signs of ovulation gotten stronger? Keep track of what's happening throughout your week and your cycles over the next three months. It's too easy to forget where we were when we're feeling really good! Give yourself a pat on the back each and every time you make a self-caring choice.

## TREAT THIS PLAN AS SELF-CARE

By treating this plan as self-care, you're sending the right messages to your inner self and your ovaries—that there is abundance, safety, and nourishment available. These are messages that signal to the body that it's an optimum time for conception and pregnancy. You can also use this time to reconnect with your partner through the grounding daily rituals of cooking and eating and simply enjoying sharing time together. Those who cook together make babies together. (I'd definitely like to see this hook played out in a subtitled European rom-com someday.)

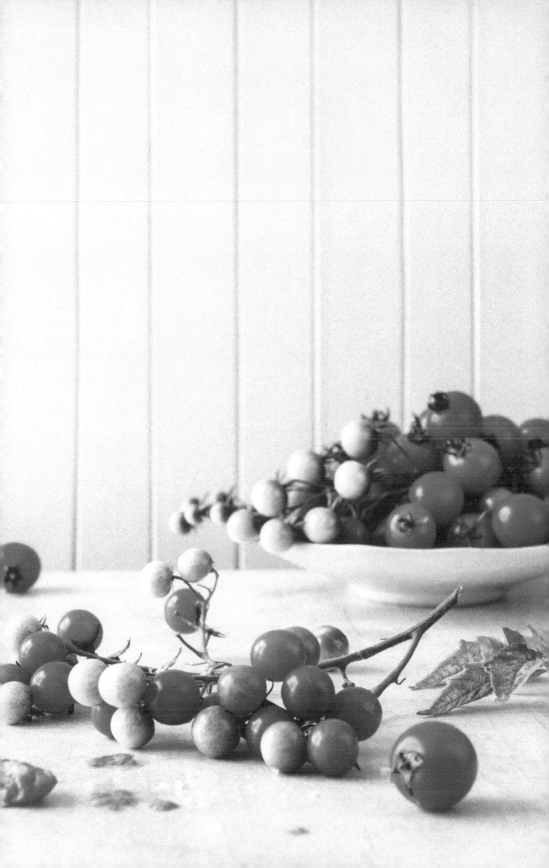

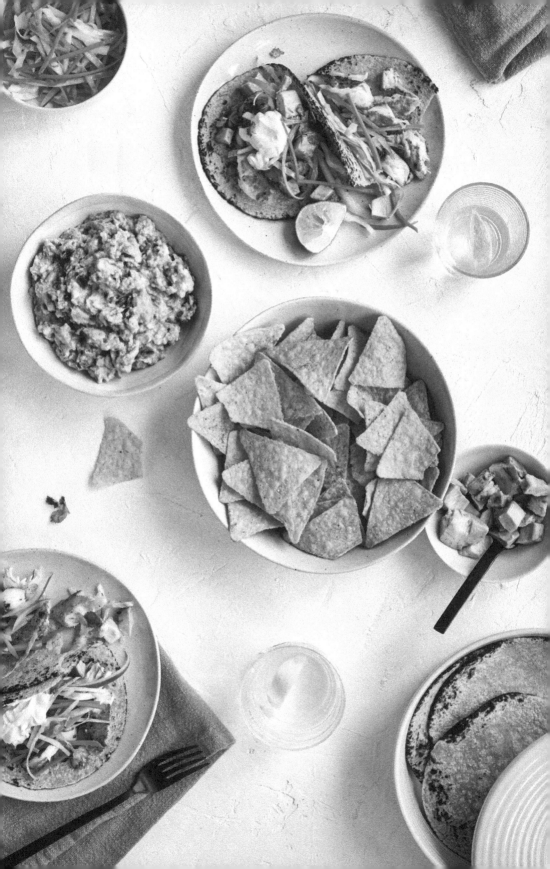

# PART THREE

# Let's Eat

# Final Words of Wisdom

Before I sign off and let you get cooking, let's check in one more time. If you're feeling any hesitation, doubt, or overwhelm in response to what I've suggested in this book, remember that the hardest thing about any course of action is to simply start. Feeling both excitement and resistance are completely natural, even if you're completely committed to increasing your chances of fertility success.

You're a unique individual, and there is no such thing as the "perfect" diet, let alone one that will solve all fertility challenges. Give yourself permission to approach this like a scientist starting an experiment: Follow the steps, and observe what happens. If there's a substitution you find that works better for you or your partner in eating for fertility, go for it. You can use the extra recipe pages in this book to keep track of variations or record additional recipes that fit the bill.

Remember, too, that as much as you're choosing to eat in a way that specifically benefits fertility, there are a whole bunch of factors influencing your fertility journey that are outside your direct control. At some point, like thousands of women going through their fertility journey, you may decide you need a change. Whether that's a change in IVF protocol, doctor, timeline, or even how you're feeling about yourself through this, know that you can use the meal plans as a resource for as long or as short a time as you'd like. It's simply a nourishing way of eating that offers plenty of health benefits even beyond egg quality and fertility. Be empowered in your fertility journey, and choose what feels right for you.

Grab a diet buddy (partners make great ones!), connect socially with other women who "get it." Community and connection are a part of all the integrative fertility programs at my clinic, and I host a private Fertility BOOSTCamp Facebook group that's free to join. Meet with your choice of health care providers until you find the right fit.

I wish you delicious success with your meal plan, your fertility journey, and long beyond!

Elizabeth Cherevaty


As a chef and educator, I'm very honored to be sharing these recipes with you, and hope you have just as much fun preparing and enjoying them as I've had creating them. When it comes to making food in your home, your creativity is what makes it unique. I encourage you to take these recipes and use them as a guide—feel free to adjust them to your individual palate and preferences. Feeling flexible with the recipes is one way to ensure that cooking and eating are both supportive to your health goals, and most importantly, delicious and fun! Go ahead, play with your food and know that happiness is homemade. Play with your food, my friend; play with your food.

Charleston F. Dollano
Executive Chef and Educator
What's Good Inc.

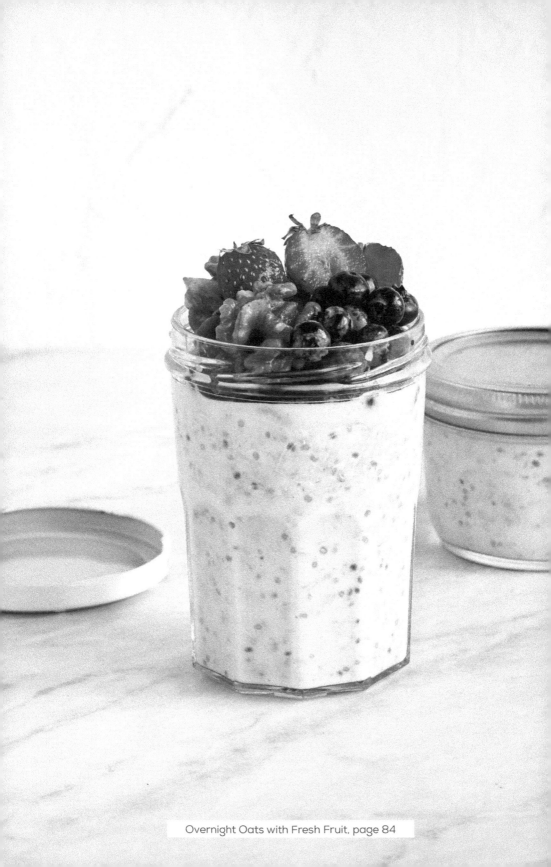

Overnight Oats with Fresh Fruit, page 84

# Breakfast

# Chocolate Monkey Smoothie

GLUTEN FREE | SERVES 2
PREP TIME: 8 MINUTES

Cacao nibs are a source of fertility-friendly antioxidants, iron, and magnesium, and they add a healthy dark chocolate flavor to all sorts of recipes. This treat counts as a wonderful breakfast or post-workout snack of champions.

2 cups baby spinach or baby kale

2 cups unsweetened almond milk

1 chopped frozen banana

½ cup unsweetened Greek or coconut yogurt

½ cup ice

3 tablespoons cacao nibs

2 tablespoons nut butter (almond, cashew, or peanut)

1 teaspoon pure maple syrup

¼ teaspoon pure vanilla extract

1. Combine the spinach, almond milk, banana, yogurt, ice, cacao nibs, nut butter, maple syrup, and vanilla in a high-powered blender, and blend on high until smooth (see tip).

2. Pour into a Mason jar. Enjoy immediately or keep chilled until ready to enjoy.

INGREDIENT TIP: If you process the smoothie just until the cacao nibs are broken up but not completely blended, you'll have a texture that simulates chocolate chips.

PER SERVING: Calories: 357; Total Fat: 19 g; Saturated Fat: 3 g; Total Carbohydrates: 33 g; Fiber: 12 g; Protein: 10 g; Sodium: 311 mg

# Tropical Green Smoothie

DAIRY FREE | GLUTEN FREE | SERVES 2
PREP TIME: 8 MINUTES

To save time in the morning, prep and assemble the ingredients for this refreshing smoothie the night before and keep them refrigerated in a Mason jar until you're ready to blend. Put the pineapple in the jar first, so its juices don't drip over the greens and wilt them. Once blended, pour your smoothie into the same jar, pop a lid on it, and go!

2 cups diced frozen or fresh pineapple

1 cup coconut milk

1 cup coconut water or water

4 leaves green or black kale, stemmed and finely chopped

3 leaves romaine lettuce, finely chopped

1 scoop vanilla protein powder

1 tablespoon coconut oil

1 teaspoon grated fresh ginger

Juice of ½ lime

1.  Combine the pineapple, coconut milk, coconut water, kale, romaine, protein powder, oil, ginger, and lime juice in a blender; process until smooth.

2.  Enjoy immediately, or pour the smoothie into a Mason jar and refrigerate until you're ready to drink it.

INGREDIENT TIP: My favorite vanilla protein powders are either collagen-based or a vegan protein combination based on pea protein. For more on protein powders, see "Fertility and Pregnancy Supplements" on page 161.

PER SERVING: Calories: 533; Total Fat: 37 g; Saturated Fat: 32 g; Total Carbohydrates: 41 g; Fiber: 6 g; Protein: 20 g; Sodium: 126 mg

# Overnight Oats with Fresh Fruit

DAIRY FREE | SERVES 2
PREP TIME: 15 MINUTES

Overnight oats take very little time to make and can be eaten cold or hot. To enjoy them hot, simply empty the contents into a pot, add ⅛ to ¼ cup additional liquid, and heat to your desired temperature.

1 cup coconut yogurt, coconut milk, or unsweetened almond milk

½ cup rolled oats

1 tablespoon white or black chia seeds

2 teaspoons pure maple syrup

4 strawberries, cut into ½-inch pieces, plus more if desired

12 blueberries, plus more if desired

4 walnut halves

Unsweetened shredded coconut (toasted), for garnish

1. In a bowl, combine the yogurt or milk, oats, chia seeds, and maple syrup.

2. In each of two Mason jars, quickly layer a quarter of the fruit and a quarter of the oat mixture. Repeat with another layer of each.

3. Cover and refrigerate overnight.

4. Uncover and top with the walnuts and coconut, as well as additional fruit if desired. Store for up to one day in the refrigerator.

**MAKE IT GLUTEN FREE:** Look for gluten-free rolled oats. Oats don't contain gluten, but they are often processed in the same facilities as wheat, barley, or rye and can become contaminated.

**VARIATION TIP:** The diversity of flavors you can incorporate is up to you. To make "apple pie" overnight oats, just add cinnamon and chopped apples or applesauce. For a dessert-like flavor, add dark chocolate chips. The possibilities are endless.

**PER SERVING:** Calories: 339; Total Fat: 17 g; Saturated Fat: 3 g; Total Carbohydrates: 42 g; Fiber: 7 g; Protein: 9 g; Sodium: 53 mg

# Avocado Toast

DAIRY FREE | VEGAN | SERVES 2
PREP TIME: 5 MINUTES | COOK TIME: 5 MINUTES

Make this light meal "comfort food" and increase the protein by serving it with ½ cup of baked beans on the side.

4 slices whole-grain bread

1 avocado, pitted, peeled, and sliced

⅛ teaspoon fine sea salt

⅛ teaspoon freshly ground black pepper

Extra-virgin olive oil

1. Toast the bread.

2. Arrange one-quarter of the avocado slices on each piece of toast, then sprinkle with the salt, pepper, and a drizzle of olive oil.

**MAKE IT GLUTEN FREE:** Choose gluten-free whole-grain bread.

**INGREDIENT TIP:** Ripen firm avocados faster by placing them in a brown paper bag with an apple.

**PER SERVING:** Calories: 314; Total Fat: 16 g; Saturated Fat: 2 g; Total Carbohydrates: 35 g; Fiber: 11 g; Protein: 10 g; Sodium: 299 mg

Zucchini and Roasted Red Pepper Omelet with Avocado Toast, pages 86 and 95

# CHAPTER SIX

## Lunch and Dinner

# Salad in a Jar

DAIRY FREE | GLUTEN FREE | SERVES 1
PREP TIME: 10 MINUTES

This portable lunch option is an easy and fun way to make sure you're getting in a variety of fresh vegetables each week. Put the dressing in the jar first, so it will end up on top of your salad when you empty it into your bowl at lunchtime.

2 tablespoons Apple Cider Vinaigrette (page 134) or other salad dressing of your choice

½ cup chopped carrots

⅛ cup chopped red onion

2 hard-boiled eggs, chopped (or other cooked protein of your choice)

½ cup cooked quinoa

½ cup chopped cucumbers

1 cup fresh greens, such as baby kale, baby spinach, or chopped romaine lettuce

¼ cup Seedy Granola (page 122) or a combination of seeds and nuts, such as sliced almonds, sunflower seeds, sesame seeds, and pumpkin seeds

1. Put the salad dressing in a Mason jar, followed by the carrots and onion.

2. Layer with the eggs, quinoa, and cucumbers.

3. Add the greens, and top with the granola. Cover and refrigerate.

4. When ready to eat, invert the jar to dump the salad into a bowl. The dressing will drizzle over the other ingredients.

**MAKE IT GLUTEN FREE:** Use gluten-free oats in the Seedy Granola.

**INGREDIENT TIP:** Substitute local, in-season vegetables for the cucumbers and carrots. Add the firmest vegetables (such as carrots and onions) right after the dressing, as they will not get soggy.

**PER SERVING:** Calories: 577; Total Fat: 43 g; Saturated Fat: 13 g; Total Carbohydrates: 36 g; Fiber: 6 g; Protein: 18 g; Sodium: 260 mg

# Green Salad

DAIRY FREE (DEPENDING ON SALAD DRESSING CHOICE)

GLUTEN FREE | SERVES 2

PREP TIME: 5 MINUTES

This is the simplest of all salads to prepare. You can use any combination of fresh leafy greens—one of the richest sources of folate available. We like a mixture of prewashed baby greens such as baby spinach, baby kale, and, for a little color and interesting flavors, mesclun mix.

3 to 4 cups fresh leafy greens

2 tablespoons Apple Cider Vinaigrette (page 134) or other olive oil–based salad dressing of your choice

1. Place greens in a medium-size bowl, add the dressing, and toss gently to coat

2. Divide the salad between two bowls and serve alongside any meal.

COOKING TIP: Change it up! Add ½ cup of your favorite chopped vegetables, berries, nuts, or seeds to this staple side salad.

PER SERVING: Calories: 159; Total Fat: 13 g; Saturated Fat: 2 g; Total Carbohydrates: 12 g; Fiber: 1 g; Protein: 1 g; Sodium: 8 mg

# Caprese Salad

Good ingredients make all the difference in the outcome of a recipe. This Italian classic tastes best when made with fresh, vine-ripened tomatoes drizzled with your favorite extra-virgin olive oil.

2 ripe tomatoes, cut into ½-inch-thick slices

1 (4-ounce) ball buffalo mozzarella, cut into ½-inch-thick slices (see tip)

2 tablespoons extra-virgin olive oil

4 or 5 fresh basil leaves, for garnish

1. On two salad plates, arrange the tomato and mozzarella slices in alternating, partly overlapping layers.

2. Drizzle each salad with the oil.

3. Garnish with the basil before serving.

SUBSTITUTION TIP: If your local grocery store doesn't carry buffalo milk mozzarella—the original version of this stretchy cheese—you can substitute with fresh mozzarella made from cow's milk. If fresh basil isn't available, sprinkle the salad with a teaspoon of dried basil.

PER SERVING: Calories: 302; Total Fat: 26 g; Saturated Fat: 2 g; Total Carbohydrates: 7 g; Fiber: 2 g; Protein: 11 g; Sodium: 46 mg

# Cream of Mushroom Soup

GLUTEN FREE | SERVES 4
PREP TIME: 15 MINUTES | COOK TIME: 30 MINUTES

The beauty of this soup is that it can be made with your choice of milk and as many varieties of mushrooms as you'd like. I recommend using at least three varieties in each batch you make. The world is your oyster . . . mushroom.

¼ cup ghee or clarified butter

1 cup sliced cremini mushrooms (¼-inch-thick slices)

1 cup sliced shiitake mushrooms (¼-inch-thick slices)

1 cup finely torn oyster mushrooms

2 teaspoons garlic powder

¼ cup sliced leeks, white parts only (¼-inch-thick slices)

4 cups chicken or vegetable stock or Basic Bone Broth (page 120)

1 cup heavy (whipping) cream or full-fat coconut milk

½ teaspoon fine sea salt

1 tablespoon fresh thyme leaves or 1 teaspoon dried thyme

1. In a large pot over medium-high heat, melt the ghee or clarified butter.

2. Once the ghee is hot (after about 40 seconds), add the mushrooms and cook, stirring occasionally, until they begin to sweat.

3. Add the garlic and continue to cook, stirring occasionally, until the mushrooms are golden brown.

4. Reduce the heat to medium and add the leeks. Cook for about 3 minutes, stirring occasionally, and then add the stock.

CONTINUED >

5. Allow the stock to come to a simmer, then add the cream and continue to cook over low heat, stirring frequently, for another 10 minutes (see tip). Stir in the salt, then divide the soup among four bowls. Sprinkle each serving with some of the thyme.

6. Serve hot with a slice of crusty bread and a side salad. To increase protein content, top the salad with 2 tablespoons of seeds and nuts and a sliced boiled egg.

INGREDIENT TIP: You don't want to cook the cream or coconut milk too long, or the soup will lose the creaminess you are trying to preserve.

PER SERVING: Calories: 404; Total Fat: 37 g; Saturated Fat: 23 g; Total Carbohydrates: 11 g; Fiber: 2 g; Protein: 4 g; Sodium: 370 mg

# Zucchini and Roasted Red Pepper Omelet

## (with Veggie Western Sandwich variation)

GLUTEN FREE | SERVES 4 | PREP TIME: 20 MINUTES
COOK TIME: 10 MINUTES

This breakfast-for-dinner meal is perfect for a busy weeknight. Pasture-raised eggs are a rich source of choline, a nutrient that supports your future baby's brain development during pregnancy. Serve this dish with Avocado Toast (page 86), or keep it gluten free and wrap it in lettuce leaves or serve it on a bed of mixed greens. See the tip for a Veggie Western Sandwich variation.

8 large pasture-raised eggs

2 tablespoons chopped fresh basil

2 tablespoons chopped fresh dill

½ teaspoon fine sea salt, plus more as needed

5 tablespoons coconut oil, divided

4 jarred roasted red peppers, drained, rinsed, and chopped

1 zucchini, cut into matchsticks

8 tablespoons crumbled goat cheese

1. In a bowl, beat the eggs. Stir in the basil, dill, and salt, and set aside.

2. In a medium skillet over medium heat, heat 2 tablespoons of the oil. Add the peppers and zucchini, and sauté just until the zucchini gets soft. Transfer the vegetable mixture to a plate.

3. Return the skillet to the stove over medium-high heat. Once the skillet is hot, add the remaining 3 tablespoons of coconut oil, and swish it around to coat the entire bottom of the skillet.

**CONTINUED >**

4. Pour the egg mixture into the skillet. With a spatula, lift the corner of the eggs to let the uncooked eggs trickle underneath. Flip once and continue cooking without stirring until cooked and fluffy.

5. Spoon the vegetable mixture and the goat cheese on top of the cooked eggs. Using a spatula, gently fold the eggs in half over the filling, cover the skillet, and allow the cheese to melt.

6. When the eggs are no longer runny, remove the skillet from heat. Cut the omelet into four wedges, and transfer the wedges to individual plates. Serve with avocado toast on the side.

VARIATION TIP: To prepare a veggie-boosted version of the classic "Western Sandwich," prepare the omelet as directed, reserving two of the quartered omelet sections. Reheat one wedge of omelet in a skillet over medium-low heat for 5 minutes per side, or heat it on a plate in the microwave for 30 to 60 seconds. Place the heated omelet on a slice of toast or fresh bread, top with a slice of fresh tomato and your favorite leafy green, and enjoy!

PER SERVING: Calories: 374; Total Fat: 29 g; Saturated Fat: 20 g; Total Carbohydrates: 14 g; Fiber: 2 g; Protein: 17 g; Sodium: 484 mg

# Scallop and Broccoli Stir-Fry

DAIRY FREE | GLUTEN FREE | SERVES 4
PREP TIME: 10 MINUTES | COOK TIME: 15 MINUTES

This recipe uses broccoli and sesame seeds, which are among the foods richest in calcium, and a savory tamari sauce, but you can get creative with any sauce or add-ins you like (see tip). Enjoy this dish over brown rice, quinoa, or millet.

3 tablespoons coconut oil

½ cup thinly sliced shallots

4 cups chopped broccoli florets (½-inch pieces)

1 cup chopped asparagus (1-inch pieces)

1 teaspoon garlic powder

1 pound baby bay scallops, fresh or frozen

2 tablespoons tamari

1 teaspoon sesame oil

⅛ teaspoon red pepper flakes

¼ cup sesame seeds, for garnish

1. In a large skillet or wok, heat the oil over medium-high heat.

2. Add the shallots and cook, stirring occasionally, until translucent.

3. Add the broccoli to the pan and cook, stirring frequently, for about 4 minutes, then add the asparagus. Allow some crowding in the pan, as that will create steam and the vegetables will cook in their own juices. Test the vegetables with a fork every few minutes. When they are tender-crisp, add the garlic powder and stir well.

4. Add the scallops and cook, stirring occasionally, just until the scallops firm up and become opaque.

CONTINUED >

5. Add the tamari, sesame oil, and pepper flakes. Toss until evenly coated.

6. Garnish with the sesame seeds, and serve over cooked whole grains.

SUBSTITUTION TIP: Instead of tamari, change up the flavors with a premade teriyaki or sweet and sour sauce, or go au naturel with no sauce and let the vegetables and protein complement each other. If you like, swap in diced chicken breast or shrimp as the protein in this dish.

STORAGE TIP: Cooked stir-fry can be refrigerated in a covered container for up to 2 days. Reheated scallops may turn tough, so pick them out before reheating, and once the vegetables are hot, add them back in for about 5 minutes on the stove over medium heat (or 30 seconds in the microwave).

PER SERVING: Calories: 309; Total Fat: 17 g; Saturated Fat: 10 g; Total Carbohydrates: 17 g; Fiber: 4 g; Protein: 26 g; Sodium: 642 mg

# Blackened Fish Tacos

DAIRY FREE | GLUTEN FREE | SERVES 3
PREP TIME: 20 MINUTES | COOK TIME: 5 MINUTES

Fish tacos made me appreciate seafood's textures and flavors. They can be made with any type of fish you like (this recipe uses black cod), and they can be battered, grilled, or, in this case, blackened. Blackening allows you to enjoy a little bit of both the battered and grilled sensations. The rub on the fish turns somewhat crispy with a hint of smoke, similar to that achieved on a grill.

## FOR THE DRY RUB

1 tablespoon paprika

1½ teaspoons ground turmeric

1½ teaspoons ground coriander

1½ teaspoons coarsely ground black pepper

½ teaspoon ground ginger

¼ teaspoon ground cumin

½ teaspoon mustard powder

¼ teaspoon cayenne pepper, more or less as desired

## FOR THE TOPPINGS

1 avocado, pitted, peeled, and diced

3 tablespoons extra-virgin olive oil

½ teaspoon fine sea salt

3 cups prepared coleslaw mix

2 tablespoons red wine vinaigrette or Apple Cider Vinaigrette (page 134)

½ apple, cored and cut into matchsticks

3 corn tortillas

Coconut yogurt, for garnish

3 lime wedges, for garnish

CONTINUED >

**Blackened Fish Tacos** CONTINUED

3 (4-ounce) black cod
(or tilapia or rock fish) fillets

½ teaspoon fine sea salt

¼ cup coconut oil

In a small bowl, combine the paprika, turmeric, coriander, black pepper, ginger, cumin, mustard powder, and cayenne, and mix well. Set aside.

1. In a bowl, combine the avocado, olive oil, and salt. Mix together, cover, and set aside in the refrigerator.

2. In another bowl, combine the coleslaw mix and red wine vinaigrette, and use clean hands to massage the cabbage to your desired texture. Mix in the apples, cover, and set aside in the refrigerator.

1. Dab the fish fillets with a paper towel to remove any excess moisture, and season with the salt.

2. Sprinkle a little bit of the rub in the bottom of a shallow dish, then place the fillets on top. Sprinkle more rub on top of the fillets, and move them around so they are completely covered with rub.

3.  Place a large skillet over medium-high heat. Once the pan is very hot, add the coconut oil and let it melt.

4.  Add the fish to the hot skillet. Once the edges of the fillets are golden brown and the fish is half white and half translucent, flip the fillets and continue cooking until the fish is completely white and no longer translucent, 5 to 8 minutes total. Avoid overcooking.

5.  Warm the tortillas for a few seconds, either in the microwave, covered with a damp paper towel, or in the pan with no oil added.

6.  Place the fish fillets on top of the corn tortillas. Top as desired. Sprinkle with lime juice and enjoy.

STORAGE TIP: The avocado browns quickly, but in a pinch you can store your avocado, coleslaw, and fish in airtight containers in the refrigerator for up to 2 days.

VARIATION TIP: If you have any leftover tortillas, you can always make them into Taco Chips (page 130) and enjoy them with some Zesty Guacamole (page 136).

PER SERVING: Calories: 688; Total Fat: 57 g; Saturated Fat: 24 g; Total Carbohydrates: 30 g; Fiber: 9 g; Protein: 19 g; Sodium: 1,014 mg

# Dill Baked Salmon

DAIRY FREE | GLUTEN FREE | SERVES 2
PREP TIME: 5 MINUTES | COOK TIME: 15 TO 18 MINUTES

Salmon's omega-3s make it wonderfully health-supportive. This dish takes little effort to prep and not much time to cook. The important thing to remember when baking seafood is that your cooking vessel needs a lid to conserve as much moisture as possible. You can also cook the salmon wrapped in parchment paper. Enjoy this decadent dish with some baked sweet potato fries and a fresh Green Salad (page 91).

2 (5-ounce) fillets wild-caught Pacific or sockeye salmon

¼ teaspoon fine sea salt

6 sprigs fresh dill, divided

12 capers

½ lemon, sliced

3 tablespoons extra-virgin olive oil or ghee

1. Preheat the oven to 350°F. Line a casserole dish with parchment paper.

2. Place the salmon in the casserole dish. Season the salmon with the salt, then top each fillet with four sprigs of dill and half of the capers and lemon slices.

3. Drizzle the oil over the salmon.

4. Cover and bake for 15 to 18 minutes, until the fish is opaque in the center.

5. Garnish with the remaining dill. Refrigerate leftovers in an airtight container for up to 2 days.

INGREDIENT TIP: As farmed salmon contains less beneficial omega-3s and more contaminants than wild-caught species, choose wild-caught Pacific or sockeye salmon for this recipe.

PER SERVING: Calories: 378; Total Fat: 27 g; Saturated Fat: 5 g; Total Carbohydrates: 0 g; Fiber: 0 g; Protein: 33 g; Sodium: 438 mg

# Beanless Turkey Chili

DAIRY FREE | GLUTEN FREE | SERVES 8
PREP TIME: 15 MINUTES | COOK TIME: 6 HOURS

Chili could be considered a very hearty soup. I always recommend making enough for leftovers.

3 tablespoons coconut oil

3 pounds ground turkey

2 cups finely diced
white onion

1 cup finely diced
red bell pepper

1 cup finely diced zucchini

¾ cup finely diced celery

3 tablespoons chili powder

3 teaspoons garlic powder

2 teaspoons ground cumin

Fine sea salt

4 cups chicken or
vegetable stock

1 (15-ounce) can
diced tomatoes

1 (15-ounce) can
crushed tomatoes

1. In a large skillet over medium-high heat, melt the coconut oil. Add the turkey and cook, stirring and breaking apart large chunks, until the meat is browned and no longer translucent. Transfer the turkey to a slow cooker.

2. Add the onion, pepper, zucchini, and celery to the warm skillet. Stir in the chili powder, garlic powder, cumin, and salt, and sauté until the onion is translucent, about 5 minutes.

3. Scrape the vegetable mixture into the slow cooker with the turkey, and add the stock and tomatoes.

4. Cook on low for 6 hours. Serve hot.

VARIATION TIP: You can serve your chili over cooked brown rice or quinoa. I like mine topped with diced avocado or a fried egg.

PER SERVING: Calories: 295; Total Fat: 9 g; Saturated Fat: 5 g;
Total Carbohydrates: 13 g; Fiber: 4 g; Protein: 42 g; Sodium: 239 mg

# Turkey Meatballs

DAIRY FREE | MAKES 24 MEATBALLS
PREP TIME: 10 MINUTES | COOK TIME: 15 TO 20 MINUTES

Meatballs can be made with any type of ground meat. Our recipe uses turkey because it is rich in amino acids and tryptophan, which supplies a needed building block for the feel-good neurotransmitter, serotonin. Fertility nutrition research also suggests that poultry is a better choice than red meat, so we've taken this traditional favorite and turkey-fied it!

1 pound ground turkey

1 cup chopped kale

½ cup shredded carrots

1 large pasture-raised egg

2 tablespoons ground oats, plus more if needed

2 tablespoons coconut oil

1 tablespoon chopped fresh basil

1 teaspoon dried thyme

½ teaspoon garlic powder

½ teaspoon fine sea salt

1. Preheat the oven to 400°F. Line a rimmed baking sheet with parchment paper.

2. In a large bowl, mix together the turkey, kale, carrots, egg, oats, oil, basil, thyme, garlic powder, and salt until everything is evenly incorporated. Test to make sure you can form the mixture into balls. If it's too sticky, add a little more ground oats.

3. Roll the turkey mixture into 1- to 1 ½-inch balls, and spread them on the prepared baking sheet.

4. Bake for 15 to 20 minutes or until the meatballs are no longer pink inside.

5. Serve warm. Store leftover meatballs in an airtight container in the refrigerator for up to 3 days.

**MAKE IT GLUTEN FREE:** Choose gluten-free oats.

**VARIATION TIP:** Keep leftover meatballs in the freezer, then reheat and serve them with rice or noodles. You can also make a hot turkey meatball sandwich by slicing 2 meatballs in half, reheating them, and serving them between 2 slices of bread. Complete the sandwich with lettuce, tomato, or your other favorite fixings.

**PER SERVING (6 MEATBALLS):** Calories: 229; Total Fat: 10 g; Saturated Fat: 7 g; Total Carbohydrates: 6 g; Fiber: 1 g; Protein: 29 g; Sodium: 382 mg

# Coconut Curry Chicken

DAIRY FREE | GLUTEN FREE | SERVES 8
PREP TIME: 15 MINUTES | COOK TIME: 20 MINUTES

Curry is one of those braised dishes that gets tastier over time. Marinate your meat to infuse it with an even richer curry flavor. Enjoy this dish over rice with a side salad.

2 pounds boneless, skinless chicken breasts or thighs, cut into 1-inch pieces

½ tablespoon curry powder

½ tablespoon plus ½ teaspoon fine sea salt, divided

3 tablespoons coconut oil

2 cups finely diced white onion

1 tablespoon ground ginger

½ tablespoon garlic powder

2 (13.5-ounce) cans coconut milk

3 tablespoons Thai red curry paste

1½ cups frozen diced precooked squash

½ to 1 cup water or chicken stock

1 cup baby spinach

1. In a bowl, rub the chicken with the curry powder and ½ tablespoon of salt. Cover the bowl and allow the chicken to marinate for at least 15 minutes.

2. In a large pot over medium heat, melt the coconut oil. Add the onion, ginger, and garlic powder and cook, stirring frequently, until the onion is translucent.

3. Add the chicken and stir until the surface of the meat turns pale white with a hint of curry color, about 5 minutes.

4. Add the coconut milk, curry paste, and squash. Simmer over medium heat until the chicken reaches an internal temperature of 165°F.

5. Throughout the cooking process, the coconut milk may reduce and thicken. If you prefer it less thick, add a little water or chicken stock to loosen it up. Add just enough so that your curry resembles a thick sauce that can be easily poured.

6. Add the spinach and stir it in until just wilted.

7. Season with the remaining ½ teaspoon salt, and serve the curry over rice pilaf with a green salad on the side.

8. Refrigerate leftovers for up to 3 days or freeze it in individual portions for another day.

SUBSTITUTION TIP: For a sweeter curry, you can substitute the squash with the same amount of cooked, cubed yams or sweet potatoes.

PER SERVING: Calories: 411; Total Fat: 31 g; Saturated Fat: 25 g; Total Carbohydrates: 10 g; Fiber: 2 g; Protein: 26 g; Sodium: 174 mg

# Slow Cooker Pulled Chicken

DAIRY FREE | GLUTEN FREE | SERVES 6
PREP TIME: 15 MINUTES | COOK TIME: 6 HOURS

This is a great way to use any kind of meat (chicken, pork, beef, or lamb) you might have in your refrigerator or freezer. All you do is add aromatics, premade sauce, and broth, then cook the meat low and slow. Enjoy this dish with a side of coleslaw.

2 tablespoons coconut oil

1 cup diced white onion

2 pounds boneless, skinless chicken thighs or breasts

½ cup orange juice

¼ cup chicken broth

3 garlic cloves, chopped

1 tablespoon paprika

2 ¼ teaspoons chili powder

1 teaspoon ground cumin

1 teaspoon dried oregano

1 teaspoon fine sea salt

½ (15-ounce) can cannellini beans, drained and rinsed

1. In a skillet over medium heat, melt the coconut oil. Add the onion and cook, stirring occasionally, until translucent. Transfer to a slow cooker.

2. Add the chicken, orange juice, broth, garlic, paprika, chili powder, cumin, oregano, and salt to the slow cooker. Cover and cook on low for 6 hours or until the chicken shreds easily with two forks.

3. Add the beans 1 hour before the end of the cooking time (see tip).

4. Serve with a side of coleslaw.

5. If desired, you can lay out your cooked meat on a baking sheet and broil it so it becomes a little bit crispy.

6. Leftover pulled chicken can be frozen in individual portions for later use.

INGREDIENT TIP: While it's directed to add the beans closer to the end of cook time, you can also add them with the chicken if that is more convenient.

PER SERVING: Calories: 183; Total Fat: 5 g; Saturated Fat: 2 g; Total Carbohydrates: 15 g; Fiber: 4 g; Protein: 21 g; Sodium: 62 mg

# Chicken Cacciatore with Kale Caesar Salad

DAIRY FREE | GLUTEN FREE | SERVES 6
PREP TIME: 25 MINUTES | COOK TIME: 30 TO 40 MINUTES

Chicken cacciatore is a braised dish that has the perfect complex balance of salty, sweet, and bitter flavors. It's a comforting dish for cold winter nights, but it can be enjoyed in the summer with a side salad, too. When chicken is cooked on the bone, more nutrients are captured in the meal.

### FOR THE KALE CAESAR SALAD

- 1 bunch kale, washed, patted dry, stemmed, and chopped into bite-size pieces
- ⅓ cup (about 6 tablespoons) Caesar Salad Dressing (page 135)
- ½ cup croutons (optional)

### FOR THE CHICKEN CACCIATORE

- 6 bone-in, skinless chicken thighs
- Fine sea salt
- Coarsely ground black pepper
- 3 tablespoons coconut oil
- 1 large red bell pepper, seeded and julienned
- 1½ cups diced white onion
- 2 garlic cloves, crushed
- 2 teaspoons dried oregano
- 2 teaspoons dried basil, plus more for garnish
- 1 (28-ounce) can diced tomatoes
- 1 cup chicken broth
- ¼ cup drained capers
- Red pepper flakes, for garnish

Prepare the salad by placing the kale in a large bowl and pouring the dressing over top. Toss well and set aside.

## TO MAKE THE CHICKEN CACCIATORE

1. Preheat the oven to 375°F. Season the chicken with salt and pepper.

2. Heat a Dutch oven or oven-safe pot over medium-high heat. Melt the coconut oil, then add the chicken. Allow the chicken to sear, flipping it only once when the thighs are golden brown around the edges, and cook until both sides are lightly brown.

3. Once the chicken is seared, transfer it to a plate and set aside.

4. Reduce the heat to medium and add the bell pepper, onion, garlic, oregano, and basil to the Dutch oven. Cook, stirring occasionally, until the onion starts to become translucent and soft, about 5 minutes.

5. Add the tomatoes, broth, and capers, and bring to a simmer.

6. Add the chicken, cover the pot, and transfer it to the preheated oven. Allow the chicken to braise for at least 20 minutes before checking it, to prevent the release of steam.

CONTINUED >

7.  Once the chicken is fully cooked (the meat should easily fall away from the bone), remove it from the oven.

8.  Serve the chicken garnished with basil and red pepper flakes, and serve the salad in separate bowls, topped with croutons (if using).

STORAGE TIP: Refrigerate leftover chicken in an airtight container for up to 3 days, or pull the chicken off the bone and freeze it in individual freezer-safe containers.

VARIATION TIP: This versatile dish can be eaten as a stew over brown rice, or the chicken can be pulled and transformed into a nice chunky sauce served over your favorite whole-grain pasta. You can also use the bones to make Basic Bone Broth (page 120).

PER SERVING: Calories: 355; Total Fat: 21 g; Saturated Fat: 9 g; Total Carbohydrates: 17 g; Fiber: 5 g; Protein: 27 g; Sodium: 813 mg

# Barbecue Chicken with Veggie Kebabs

DAIRY FREE | GLUTEN FREE | SERVES 2
PREP TIME: 15 MINUTES | COOK TIME: 20 MINUTES

Everyone loves the grill, but vegetables can be one of the most frustrating foods to cook on it. They can be hard to flip, and they can fall through the grate. Enter, skewers! Just rotate them until the veggies are tender, and voilà! You have the perfect summer side to this barbecue chicken main. No grill? No problem—we also include directions for oven cooking.

### FOR THE BARBECUE SAUCE (SEE INGREDIENT TIP)

1 (6-ounce) can tomato paste

½ cup balsamic vinegar

7 Medjool dates, pitted and cut into small pieces

2 tablespoons Dijon mustard

1 teaspoon chili powder

½ teaspoon onion powder

½ teaspoon garlic powder

¼ teaspoon freshly ground black pepper

⅛ teaspoon fine sea salt

### FOR THE CHICKEN AND KEBABS

1 cup sliced zucchini (½-inch-thick slices)

1 cup diced bell pepper (1-inch pieces)

1 cup diced red onion (1-inch pieces)

¼ cup extra-virgin olive oil, plus more as needed

1 teaspoon dried oregano

¼ teaspoon fine sea salt, plus more as needed

¼ teaspoon freshly ground black pepper, plus more as needed

2 bone-in, skin-on chicken legs

Cooked brown rice, quinoa, or millet, for serving

**CONTINUED >**

**Barbecue Chicken with Veggie Kebabs** CONTINUED

TO MAKE THE BARBECUE SAUCE

1. In a medium pot over medium heat, combine the tomato paste, vinegar, dates, mustard, chili powder, onion powder, garlic powder, pepper, and salt.

2. Stir occasionally and cook until the mixture comes to a simmer, about 10 minutes.

3. Using a stick blender, blend the mixture until smooth. Taste and season with more salt and pepper if needed. Set aside.

TO MAKE THE CHICKEN AND KEBABS

1. In a shallow container filled with water, soak 8 to 10 flat bamboo skewers.

2. Preheat the grill on medium-high heat with the lid on. If using an oven, preheat to 400°F and line 2 rimmed baking sheets with parchment paper.

3. In a large bowl, toss together the zucchini, bell pepper, onion, oil, oregano, salt, and pepper until evenly coated.

4. Thread the vegetables onto the presoaked skewers in alternating patterns.

5. Season the chicken with salt and pepper, and rub with a little bit of oil.

6. Place the vegetable kebabs on the grill. If baking, assemble the skewers on one of the prepared baking sheets, and set the baking sheet on the middle rack of the oven. Cook until the vegetables are tender and lightly charred.

7. Place the chicken on the grill, skin-side down. If you are using your oven, place the chicken skin-side down on the second prepared baking sheet and place it in the oven. Cook for at least 10 minutes before flipping, and baste the chicken with the barbecue sauce. Baste the chicken every time you flip it, every 8 minutes, until the meat is fully cooked and the juices run clear, or until the chicken reaches an internal temperature of 165°F.

8. Serve the chicken and kebabs with your whole grain of choice.

STORAGE TIP: The vegetable kebabs can be assembled ahead of time and refrigerated for up to 48 hours before cooking. Barbecue sauce that wasn't in contact with food can be refrigerated for up to 2 weeks.

INGREDIENT TIP: You can also use a store-bought barbecue sauce. Just look for one with the least amount of refined sugar or high-fructose corn syrup, or one sweetened only with honey.

PER SERVING: Calories: 553; Total Fat: 39 g; Saturated Fat: 7 g; Total Carbohydrates: 35 g; Fiber: 4 g; Protein: 21 g; Sodium: 725 mg

# Mediterranean Kebabs

DAIRY FREE | GLUTEN FREE | SERVES 5 TO 6
PREP TIME: 15 MINUTES, PLUS 1 HOUR MARINATING TIME
COOK TIME: 15 MINUTES

Kebabs originated in Turkey, and have been adopted by many other cultures throughout the centuries. Kebabs can be made with just meat, just vegetables, or a combination of the two. If you don't have a grill, read the tip below for directions for cooking on the stovetop. This recipe is designed to make leftovers. Serve the kebabs over a bed of quinoa or brown rice, or with a side salad.

1 tablespoon garlic powder

1 teaspoon dried mint

1 teaspoon dried oregano

⅛ teaspoon red pepper flakes (optional)

2 tablespoons freshly squeezed lemon juice

1¼ pounds boneless, skinless chicken or lamb, cut in 1½-inch cubes

¼ cup extra-virgin olive oil

¼ teaspoon fine sea salt

½ teaspoon coarsely ground black pepper

1. In a shallow basin of water, soak 12 flat bamboo skewers.

2. In a large bowl, combine the garlic powder, mint, oregano, pepper flakes, if using, and lemon juice. Mix together to form a paste.

3. Add the chicken to the seasoning mixture, and use your hands to evenly coat the meat with the paste. Add the oil and toss gently to coat the chicken, then cover and refrigerate for at least 1 hour to marinate.

4. After 45 minutes of marinating time, preheat the grill, making sure is the grates are well cleaned and wiped with a little oil.

5. Remove the chicken from the refrigerator, and skewer the pieces onto the presoaked bamboo skewers.

6. Season with the salt and pepper, place the skewers on the grill, and cook them for about 15 minutes, depending on thickness. Flip them only once, if possible.

7. Serve with quinoa, brown rice, or a salad.

STORAGE TIP: Kebabs can be marinated and skewered ahead of time and kept in the refrigerator for up to 2 days. For longer storage, freeze them in individual portions so they can be pulled out for meals on busier days.

COOKING TIP: To cook these kebabs on the stovetop, prepare them as directed. Heat 2 tablespoons of coconut oil in a large skillet over medium-high heat, and cook the kebabs, flipping once or twice, until the meat is cooked through, about 10 minutes total.

PER SERVING: Calories: 222; Total Fat: 13 g; Saturated Fat: 2 g; Total Carbohydrates: 2 g; Fiber: 0 g; Protein: 24 g; Sodium: 175 mg

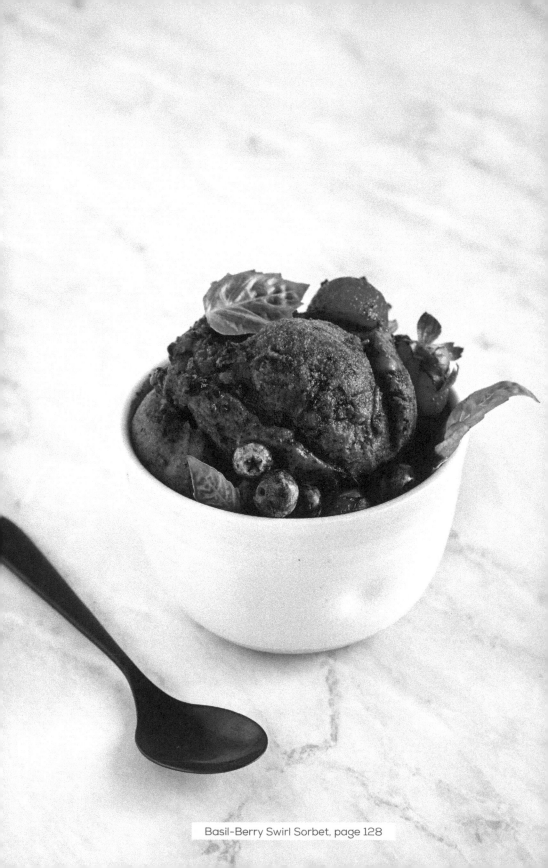

Basil-Berry Swirl Sorbet, page 128

# CHAPTER SEVEN

# Snacks

# Basic Bone Broth

DAIRY FREE | GLUTEN FREE | MAKES 4 CUPS
PREP TIME: 15 MINUTES | COOK TIME: 6 TO 12 HOURS

Bone broth is a classic foundation for savory soups, sauces, and gravies, and it can also be used to enhance flavor and nutrition when used as the cooking liquid for rice or other grains. Rich in calcium, electrolytes, and the protein known as collagen, bone broth is healing to the gut, and it can be sipped on its own at breakfast or as soothing bedtime snack. Look for the chilled broth to form a gel—a sign it's rich in the nutritious proteins collagen and gelatin. You can also add various raw vegetable "scraps" to add flavor and nutrients during the cooking time. Try carrots, cabbage, kale, and celery.

4 to 6 pieces (½ to ¾ pound total) cooked or raw bones, such as chicken, turkey, or beef

4 cups filtered water, plus more to ensure the bones are submerged in the pot

1 onion, quartered

1 garlic clove, peeled

Juice of 1 lemon

2 teaspoons fine sea salt

1 teaspoon coarsely ground black pepper

1 teaspoon dried thyme or 1 sprig fresh thyme

1 or 2 bay leaves

1. Place the bones, water, onion, garlic, lemon juice, salt, pepper, thyme, and bay leaves in a slow cooker, cover, and cook on low for 8 to 12 hours.

2. Check on the broth when it is about halfway through the cooking time; add more water if needed to fully cover all the bones.

3. Strain the broth through a colander into a large container. Discard the bones and other solids. If not serving immediately, let the broth cool, then refrigerate it in an airtight container for up to 3 days or freeze it in small containers for up to 6 months.

COOKING TIP: To prepare bone broth on the stovetop, bring all the ingredients to a boil in a large soup pot, then cover and simmer on low heat for 4 to 6 hours, adding extra water if needed to keep the bones submerged.

PER SERVING: Calories: 40; Total Fat: 1 g; Saturated Fat: 1 g; Total Carbohydrates: 4 g; Fiber: 1 g; Protein: 6 g; Sodium: 630 mg

# Seedy Granola

DAIRY FREE | VEGAN | MAKES 3½ CUPS
PREP TIME: 5 MINUTES | COOK TIME: 20 MINUTES

Granola is one of those grab-and-go snacks that can prevent blood sugar drops. It can also be enjoyed at breakfast on top of yogurt or fruit. Try making granola with any combination of seeds, nuts, and grains you like. I've chosen to feature pumpkin seeds, flaxseed, and chia seeds for their fertility-friendly nutrients and flavor. Keep in mind that humidity plays a role in granola's texture. After removing the mixture from the oven, I let it fully "dehydrate" by leaving it uncovered overnight. You may need to play with the ratio of wet ingredients at different times of the year to keep your granola nice and crunchy.

1 cup unsweetened
  shredded coconut

½ cup gluten-free rolled oats

½ cup pumpkin seeds

½ cup sunflower seeds

¼ cup chopped pecans

¼ cup sliced almonds

1 tablespoon chia seeds

1 tablespoon flaxseed

½ teaspoon fine sea salt

¼ cup melted coconut oil

¼ cup pure maple syrup

½ teaspoon pure
  vanilla extract

1. Preheat the oven to 275°F. Line a rimmed baking sheet with parchment paper.

2. In a large bowl, combine the coconut, oats, pumpkin and sunflower seeds, pecans, almonds, chia seeds, flaxseed, and salt; set aside.

3. In another bowl, whisk together the coconut oil, maple syrup, and vanilla.

4. Add the wet ingredients to the dry ingredients and mix well (see tip).

5. Spread the granola mixture on the prepared baking sheet to make an even, 1-inch-thick layer.

6. Bake for about 20 minutes, checking every 5 minutes to see if the granola has dried but not burned.

7. After the granola is baked, remove the tray from the oven and allow it to cool for 5 to 10 minutes.

8. Break the granola into chunks, then enjoy it on its own or add it to yogurt or fresh fruit. Store dry, cooled granola in an airtight container away from humidity and sunlight.

MAKE IT GLUTEN FREE: Choose gluten-free oats.

COOKING TIP: Check the consistency of your mixture at step 4. There should be enough wet ingredients to just coat all the dried ingredients. It shouldn't be swimming in the liquid.

PER SERVING (¼ CUP): Calories: 228; Total Fat: 20 g; Saturated Fat: 8 g; Total Carbohydrates: 11 g; Fiber: 3 g; Protein: 4 g; Sodium: 86 mg

# Maple Toasted Trail Mix

DAIRY FREE | GLUTEN FREE | VEGAN | MAKES 4½ CUPS
PREP TIME: 5 MINUTES | COOK TIME: 10 TO 15 MINUTES

Store-bought trail mix can contain added sugar and preservatives. This mix is a healthy make-ahead snack to keep on hand at home and work.

2 teaspoons melted coconut oil

2½ tablespoons pure maple syrup

1 teaspoon pure vanilla extract

¾ teaspoon ground cinnamon

½ teaspoon fine sea salt

1 cup raw almonds

1 cup raw pecans

1 cup raw walnuts

¾ cup unsweetened shredded coconut

¼ cup dried blueberries

¼ cup pitted Medjool dates, quartered

1. Preheat the oven to 350°F and set a rack in the middle of the oven. Line a rimmed baking sheet with parchment paper.

2. In a large bowl, whisk together the coconut oil, maple syrup, vanilla, cinnamon, and salt. Add the almonds, pecans, and walnuts to the bowl, and mix until the nuts are evenly coated. Add the coconut and mix until it is evenly incorporated.

3. Spread the mixture in a single layer on the prepared baking sheet.

4. Bake for at least 10 minutes or until the surface of the nuts is no longer sticky, checking every 3 minutes to prevent burning.

5. Once the nuts are evenly dry and toasted, remove them from the oven and let them cool for at least 10 minutes before handling.

6. In a large bowl, combine the blueberries, dates, and toasted nut mixture. Toss gently until evenly mixed. This trail mix will keep in an airtight container at room temperature for up to 2 weeks.

COOKING TIP: Let the trail mix cool completely before storing to ensure that the nuts stay crispy.

PER SERVING (¼ CUP): Calories: 176; Total Fat: 15 g; Saturated Fat: 4 g; Total Carbohydrates: 7 g; Fiber: 3 g; Protein: 4 g; Sodium: 52 mg

# Strawberry-Mango Compote

DAIRY FREE | GLUTEN FREE | SERVES 4
PREP TIME: 5 MINUTES | COOK TIME: 30 MINUTES

Saucy, fruity, and delicious, compote can almost be mistaken for but is not as thick as jam. You can make your compote chunky or smooth. If you prefer it to be smooth, simply purée it in a blender. Use this compote as a topping for yogurt or add some chopped nuts or a dollop of whipped cream (made from grass-fed heavy cream or coconut cream) for a decadent and fertility-friendly dessert.

1 pound frozen
  chopped mango

1 pound frozen strawberries

Zest and juice of
  ½ lemon, divided

¼ cup water

¼ cup honey (optional)

2 tablespoons collagen
  or gelatin powder

1 teaspoon pure
  vanilla extract

1. In a medium pot over medium-low heat, combine the mango, strawberries, lemon juice, water, honey, if using, and gelatin powder.

2. Bring the mixture to a simmer and cook for 20 minutes, stirring occasionally. The fruit will bubble, slowly turn translucent, and eventually resemble a textured syrup.

3. Stir in the vanilla extract and lemon zest. Taste and adjust the sweetness if desired.

COOKING TIP: When chilled, the compote will thicken, especially if you've added gelatin powder. With collagen powder, the compote will have a thinner consistency.

PER SERVING: Calories: 123; Total Fat: 1 g; Saturated Fat: 0 g; Total Carbohydrates: 27 g; Fiber: 4 g; Protein: 4 g; Sodium: 10 mg

# Fresh Berries and Cream

GLUTEN FREE | SERVES 2

PREP TIME: 10 TO 15 MINUTES

When berries are in season, you'll want to take advantage of this dessert that combines their juicy sweetness with cream. You can make the whipped cream with either grass-fed heavy (whipping) cream or coconut milk.

½ cup blueberries

¼ cup raspberries

¼ cup blackberries

½ cup grapes

3 fresh mint leaves, chopped

1 cup grass-fed heavy (whipping) cream or 1 (13.5-ounce) can coconut milk

¼ cup chopped nuts of choice or Seedy Granola (page 122) (optional)

1. Mix the blueberries, raspberries, blackberries, grapes, and mint in a bowl. Set aside.

2. If using the grass-fed cream, pour the cream into a bowl and whisk it until it holds stiff peaks.

3. If using the coconut milk, refrigerate the can for at least one hour, then remove it from the refrigerator and flip it upside down. Open the can, remove the coconut water for another use, and whip the thick coconut cream with a whisk in a chilled bowl until fluffy.

4. Divide the berries between two bowls, then scoop the whipped cream on top. For added texture, sprinkle with nuts or Seedy Granola. Serve immediately.

INGREDIENT TIP: Don't overwhip your whipped cream, or you'll end up making butter! If the cream starts to turn yellowish, you've gone too far.

PER SERVING: Calories: 462; Total Fat: 44 g; Saturated Fat: 27 g; Total Carbohydrates: 16 g; Fiber: 3 g; Protein: 3 g; Sodium: 46 mg

# Basil-Berry Swirl Sorbet

DAIRY FREE | GLUTEN FREE | MAKES ABOUT 7 CUPS
PREP TIME: 5 MINUTES, PLUS FREEZE TIME

The beautiful thing about this sorbet is its natural simplicity. You can purée the berries all together, or, if you want to get really gourmet, you can purée the blueberries and strawberries separately and make swirls.

3 cups frozen blueberries

2 cups frozen strawberries

Leaves from ½ bunch fresh basil, minced, plus extra leaves for garnish

2 cups full-fat, unsweetened coconut milk yogurt

Fresh berries, for garnish

1. Using a food processor or blender, purée the berries and basil until the mixture resembles shaved ice.

2. Remove about one-third of the mixture and set it aside. Add the yogurt to the food processor and purée until smooth.

3. Pour the yogurt mixture into a deep freezer-safe casserole dish, and spread it out evenly.

4. Pour the remaining berry mixture over the yogurt mixture.

5. Using a large spoon, gently swirl the berry mixture through the pan to achieve your desired look.

6. For a soft serve texture, spoon the mixture into bowls, garnish each serving with berries and a basil leaf, and enjoy right away. For a sorbet-like texture, freeze for up to one hour. Remove from the freezer 15 minutes before garnishing and serving.

PER SERVING (1 CUP): Calories: 123; Total Fat: 1 g; Saturated Fat: 1 g; Total Carbohydrates: 29 g; Fiber: 4 g; Protein: 1 g; Sodium: 30 mg

# Chia Chocolate Pudding

DAIRY FREE | GLUTEN FREE | SERVES 4

PREP TIME: 5 MINUTES, PLUS 3 HOURS RESTING TIME

This treat is a healthy but still yummy alternative to snack-pack-style chocolate puddings.

1½ cups unsweetened almond milk or coconut milk

4 tablespoons pure maple syrup or honey

2 tablespoons raw cacao powder

½ teaspoon vanilla extract

½ cup chia seeds

1. In a mixing bowl, whisk together the milk, maple syrup, cacao powder, and vanilla. Taste the mixture and adjust for sweetness with more maple syrup if needed, then whisk the mixture until smooth.

2. Add the chia seeds and stir until the mixture starts to thicken and is evenly combined.

3. Transfer the pudding to a Mason jar, and refrigerate for at least 3 hours or overnight.

4. Serve in dessert bowls.

VARIATION TIP: Layer the finished pudding with Strawberry-Mango Compote (page 126) in a Mason jar, and keep it chilled until ready to eat for a beautiful, healthy, on-the-go treat.

PER SERVING: Calories. 235; Total Fat: 11 g; Saturated Fat: 2 g; Total Carbohydrates: 30 g; Fiber: 13 g; Protein: 6 g; Sodium: 72 mg

# Taco Chips

DAIRY FREE | GLUTEN FREE | SERVES 4
PREP TIME: 10 MINUTES

Unlike many store-bought varieties, these chips are not fried with hydrogenated cooking oils, so dip away!

4 corn tortillas

2 tablespoons olive oil

⅛ teaspoon fine sea salt

1. Preheat the oven to 375°F.

2. Brush each tortilla with olive oil until they are all equally and evenly coated. Sprinkle the tortillas with the salt.

3. Stack the tortillas on top of each other, and cut them into 6 or 8 triangles (similar to a pizza).

4. Arrange the triangles on a baking sheet in a single layer; bake for 6 to 8 minutes or until crispy. (Be sure to check them after 5 minutes, as tortilla chips tend to brown pretty quickly).

5. Once your chips are done, take them out of the oven and allow them to cool and crisp before enjoying.

6. Serve with hummus or guacamole.

PER SERVING: Calories: 112; Total Fat: 8 g; Saturated Fat: 1 g; Total Carbohydrates: 11 g; Fiber: 2 g; Protein: 1 g; Sodium: 42 mg

Zesty Guacamole, page 136

# CHAPTER EIGHT

# Dressings and Dips

# Apple Cider Vinaigrette

DAIRY FREE | GLUTEN FREE | SERVES 2
PREP TIME: 5 MINUTES

Apple cider vinegar is slightly milder than white vinegar, but you can try any vinegar you like in this recipe, including balsamic, red wine, or white wine vinegars. You can also try freshly squeezed lemon or lime juice instead of vinegar. Get creative!

¼ cup extra-virgin olive oil

¼ cup apple cider vinegar

1 tablespoon honey or pure maple syrup

½ teaspoon freshly ground black pepper

¼ teaspoon dried oregano

¼ teaspoon dried thyme

⅛ teaspoon fine sea salt

1. In a small Mason jar, combine the oil, vinegar, and honey or maple syrup. Stir gently to combine, then add the pepper, oregano, thyme, and salt. Seal the jar and shake well.

2. Divide the dressing between two salads just before serving.

STORAGE TIP: This dressing will keep in the refrigerator for up to 1 week, but you'll want to remove it from the fridge an hour before eating to let the olive oil "melt."

TIME-SAVING TIP: Double the recipe and reserve two servings of dressing for your next green salad or Salad in a Jar (page 90).

PER SERVING: Calories: 257; Total Fat: 25 g; Saturated Fat: 4 g; Total Carbohydrates: 10 g; Fiber: 0 g; Protein: 0 g; Sodium: 14 mg

# Caesar Salad Dressing

DAIRY FREE | GLUTEN FREE | SERVES 4
PREP TIME: 10 MINUTES

Yes, you can buy Caesar dressing, or even a bag of ready-to-assemble Caesar salad with that plastic baggie of dressing, but why not be the boss of your body by making your own? You'll know exactly what went into it, and it will taste so much better.

1 cup avocado oil mayonnaise (see tip for vegan option)

¼ cup freshly squeezed lemon juice

3 anchovies (see tip for vegan option)

1¼ tablespoons Dijon mustard

½ teaspoon garlic purée

¼ teaspoon freshly ground black pepper

Using a food processor or stick blender, blend the mayonnaise, lemon juice, anchovies, mustard, garlic, and pepper to your desired smoothness (see cooking tip). Refrigerate in a sealed container for up to 5 days.

MAKE IT VEGAN: Omit the avocado oil mayonnaise and anchovies, and replace them with 1 cup plain, unsweetened coconut milk yogurt and 2 tablespoons drained capers.

COOKING TIP: The dressing doesn't have to be smooth. If you want a little more texture, blend it a little less. It doesn't hurt to have chunky anchovies or capers in your salad.

PER SERVING: Calories: 398; Total Fat: 42 g; Saturated Fat: 7 g; Total Carbohydrates: 1 g; Fiber: 0 g; Protein: 5 g; Sodium: 671 mg

# Zesty Guacamole

DAIRY FREE | GLUTEN FREE | VEGAN | SERVES 2
PREP TIME: 15 MINUTES

Avocados are filled with nutrition. The trick to enjoying them is twofold: (1) Serve them when they are perfectly ripe and vibrant green (see tip) and (2) mash them to your heart's content. Pair this guac with Taco Chips (page 130), use it as a topping for your favorite sandwich, or enjoy it as a dip for fresh veggies.

2 pitted and peeled avocados

1 tablespoon extra-virgin olive oil

3 tablespoons diced red onion

1½ tablespoons diced sun-dried tomato

1 tablespoon chopped fresh cilantro

⅛ teaspoon lime zest

1 tablespoon freshly squeezed lime juice

¼ teaspoon fine sea salt

1. In a large bowl, combine the avocados and oil, and mash to your desired consistency.

2. Add the onion, tomato, cilantro, and lime zest and juice, and mix until evenly incorporated.

3. Add the salt and mix until evenly distributed. Adjust the seasonings to taste, and serve with tortilla chips.

STORAGE TIP: Place your leftover guacamole in a storage container, and drizzle the surface with 1 to 2 tablespoons lime juice. This will prevent your guacamole from oxidizing too quickly.

PER SERVING: Calories: 372; Total Fat: 34 g; Saturated Fat: 5 g; Total Carbohydrates: 19 g; Fiber: 13 g; Protein: 4 g; Sodium: 320 mg

# Creamy Hummus

DAIRY FREE | GLUTEN FREE | VEGAN | SERVES 8
PREP TIME: 20 MINUTES

This savory Mediterranean spread is rich in calcium, protein, fiber, and, of course, olive oil! It makes a satisfying snack dip for veggie sticks or spread for whole-grain crackers, a wrap, crusty bread, or grilled kebabs.

½ cup tahini

¼ cup freshly squeezed lemon juice

1 garlic clove, coarsely chopped

¼ cup water

1 (15-ounce) can chickpeas, drained and rinsed

2 tablespoons extra-virgin olive oil, plus ¼ cup for garnish

½ teaspoon ground cumin

¼ teaspoon fine sea salt

¼ teaspoon paprika, for garnish

1. In a food processor or blender, combine the tahini, lemon juice, and garlic. Process until the mixture forms a paste, scraping down the sides of the processor as needed.

2. Add the water, 2 tablespoons at a time, pulsing until the mixture is smooth.

3. Add the chickpeas, 2 tablespoons of oil, and the cumin. Blend the ingredients until the mixture reaches your desired smoothness, scraping down the sides of the bowl as needed. If the hummus is too thick, you can add a little more water. Add the salt and stir to combine.

4. Transfer the hummus into a bowl, and garnish with the remaining ¼ cup of oil and paprika before serving.

PER SERVING: Calories: 179; Total Fat: 13 g; Saturated Fat: 2 g; Total Carbohydrates: 13 g; Fiber: 4 g; Protein: 6 g; Sodium: 95 mg

# WRITE-IN PLANNING PAGES

## DAY 1

BREAKFAST:

LUNCH:

DINNER:

## DAY 2

BREAKFAST:

LUNCH:

DINNER:

## DAY 3

BREAKFAST:

LUNCH:

DINNER:

## DAY 4

BREAKFAST:

LUNCH:

DINNER:

# DAY 5

BREAKFAST:
LUNCH:
DINNER:

# DAY 6

BREAKFAST:
LUNCH:
DINNER:

# DAY 7

BREAKFAST:
LUNCH:
DINNER:

## DAY 1

BREAKFAST:
LUNCH:
DINNER:

## DAY 2

BREAKFAST:
LUNCH:
DINNER:

## DAY 3

BREAKFAST:
LUNCH:
DINNER:

## DAY 4

BREAKFAST:
LUNCH:
DINNER:

## DAY 5

BREAKFAST:
LUNCH:
DINNER:

## DAY 6

BREAKFAST:
LUNCH:
DINNER:

## DAY 7

BREAKFAST:
LUNCH:
DINNER:

# DAY 1

BREAKFAST:
LUNCH:
DINNER:

# DAY 2

BREAKFAST:
LUNCH:
DINNER:

# DAY 3

BREAKFAST:
LUNCH:
DINNER:

# DAY 4

BREAKFAST:
LUNCH:
DINNER:

## DAY 5

BREAKFAST:
LUNCH:
DINNER:

## DAY 6

BREAKFAST:
LUNCH:
DINNER:

## DAY 7

BREAKFAST:
LUNCH:
DINNER:

## DAY 1

BREAKFAST:
LUNCH:
DINNER:

## DAY 2

BREAKFAST:
LUNCH:
DINNER:

## DAY 3

BREAKFAST:
LUNCH:
DINNER:

## DAY 4

BREAKFAST:
LUNCH:
DINNER:

## DAY 5

BREAKFAST:
LUNCH:
DINNER:

## DAY 6

BREAKFAST:
LUNCH:
DINNER:

## DAY 7

BREAKFAST:
LUNCH:
DINNER:

# DAY 1

BREAKFAST:
LUNCH:
DINNER:

# DAY 2

BREAKFAST:
LUNCH:
DINNER:

# DAY 3

BREAKFAST:
LUNCH:
DINNER:

# DAY 4

BREAKFAST:
LUNCH:
DINNER:

# DAY 5

BREAKFAST:
LUNCH:
DINNER:

# DAY 6

BREAKFAST:
LUNCH:
DINNER:

# DAY 7

BREAKFAST:
LUNCH:
DINNER:

## DAY 1

BREAKFAST:

LUNCH:

DINNER:

## DAY 2

BREAKFAST:

LUNCH:

DINNER:

## DAY 3

BREAKFAST:

LUNCH:

DINNER:

## DAY 4

BREAKFAST:

LUNCH:

DINNER:

# DAY 5

BREAKFAST:
LUNCH:
DINNER:

# DAY 6

BREAKFAST:
LUNCH:
DINNER:

# DAY 7

BREAKFAST:
LUNCH:
DINNER:

# DAY 1

BREAKFAST:
LUNCH:
DINNER:

# DAY 2

BREAKFAST:
LUNCH:
DINNER:

# DAY 3

BREAKFAST:
LUNCH:
DINNER:

# DAY 4

BREAKFAST:
LUNCH:
DINNER:

# DAY 5

BREAKFAST:

LUNCH:

DINNER:

# DAY 6

BREAKFAST:

LUNCH:

DINNER:

# DAY 7

BREAKFAST:

LUNCH:

DINNER:

# DAY 1

BREAKFAST:
LUNCH:
DINNER:

# DAY 2

BREAKFAST:
LUNCH:
DINNER:

# DAY 3

BREAKFAST:
LUNCH:
DINNER:

# DAY 4

BREAKFAST:
LUNCH:
DINNER:

# DAY 5

BREAKFAST:
LUNCH:
DINNER:

# DAY 6

BREAKFAST:
LUNCH:
DINNER:

# DAY 7

BREAKFAST:
LUNCH:
DINNER:

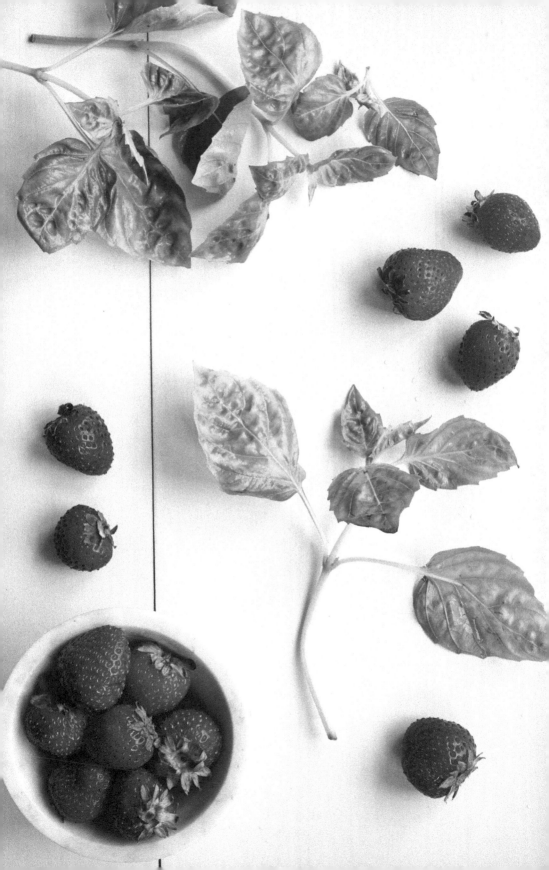

# GLOSSARY OF MEDICAL ABBREVIATIONS

Here are the most common abbreviations you will encounter in online forums and articles and in your practitioner's notes throughout your IVF journey. Use this list as a handy cheat sheet whenever you are stumped by the often dizzying medical speak surrounding this very personal time of your life.

**AH:** assisted hatching

**AI:** artificial insemination

**AMH:** anti-mullerian hormone

**ANA:** anti-nuclear antibody

**Anti-TG:** anti-thyroglobulin antibody

**Anti-TPO:** anti-thyroperoxidase antibody

**aPL:** anti-phospholipid antibody

**APS:** anti-phospholipid syndrome

**ART:** assisted reproductive technology

**ASA:** anti-sperm antibody

**BBT:** basal body temperature

**BMI:** body mass index

**CD:** cycle day

**DI:** donor insemination

**DNA:** deoxyribonucleic acid, or genes/genetic material

**DOR:** diminished ovarian reserve

**DPI:** days post-insemination

**DPO:** days post-ovulation

**DPR:** days post-retrieval

**DPT:** days post-transfer

**E2:** estradiol

**EMB:** endometrial biopsy

**ER:** egg retrieval

**ET:** embryo transfer

**FET:** frozen embryo transfer

**FHR:** fetal heart rate

**FSH:** follicle stimulating hormone

**HbA1C:** hemoglobin A1C

**hCG:** human chorionic gonadotropin or beta-hCG

**HOMA-IR:** an index of insulin resistance

**HSG:** hysterosalpingogram, an imaging study of the uterus and fallopian tubes using x-ray

**IM:** intramuscular (injection)

**IUGR:** intra-uterine growth retardation

**IUI:** intra-uterine insemination

**IVF:** in vitro fertilization

**IVIG:** intravenous immunoglobulin

**LAP:** laparoscopy

**LMP:** last menstrual period (start date)

**LPD:** luteal phase defect

**MESA:** microsurgical epididymal sperm aspiration

**MF:** male factor (infertility)

**MTHFR:** methylenetetrahydrofolate reductase

**O, OV:** ovulation

**OB/GYN:** obstetrician/gynecologist

**OC, OCP:** oral contraceptive (pill)

**OD:** oocyte donor, ovulatory dysfunction

**OHSS:** ovarian hyperstimulation syndrome

**OTC:** over-the-counter

**P4:** progesterone

**PCO:** polycystic ovaries

**PCOS:** polycystic ovarian syndrome

**PG:** pregnant

**PGA, PGD, PGS:** pre-implantation genetic analysis/diagnosis/ screening

**PID:** pelvic inflammatory disease

**PIO:** progesterone in oil

**POF:** premature ovarian failure

**RE:** reproductive endocrinologist

**RhFSH:** recombinant human FSH

**RPL:** recurrent pregnancy loss

**Rx:** prescription

**SA:** semen analysis

**SHG, Sono:** sonohysterogram, an imaging study of the uterus and fallopian tubes using ultrasound

**STI:** sexually transmitted infection

**SubQ:** subcutaneous (injection)

**Sx:** symptoms

**T:** testosterone

**T1DM, T2DM:** type 1 or type 2 diabetes

**T3, T4:** thyroid hormone

**TORCH:** test for toxoplasmosis, other, rubella, cytomegalo-virus, and herpes viruses

**TSH:** thyroid stimulating hormone

**TTC:** trying to conceive

**TTCAR:** trying to conceive after reversal

**US:** ultrasound

**VR:** vasectomy reversal

**WNL:** within normal limits

# THE CLEAN FIFTEEN™ AND DIRTY DOZEN™

A nonprofit environmental watchdog organization called Environmental Working Group (EWG) looks at data supplied by the US Department of Agriculture (USDA) and the Food and Drug Administration (FDA) about pesticide residues. Each year it compiles a list of the best and worst pesticide loads found in commercial crops. You can use these lists to decide which fruits and vegetables to buy organic to minimize your exposure to pesticides and which produce is considered safe enough to buy conventionally. This does not mean they are pesticide-free, though, so wash these fruits and vegetables thoroughly. The list is updated annually, and you can find it online at EWG.org/FoodNews.

## DIRTY DOZEN™

| | | | |
|---|---|---|---|
| 1. | strawberries | 7. | peaches |
| 2. | spinach | 8. | cherries |
| 3. | kale | 9. | pears |
| 4. | nectarines | 10. | tomatoes |
| 5. | apples | 11. | celery |
| 6. | grapes | 12. | potatoes |

*Additionally, nearly three-quarters of hot pepper samples contained pesticide residues.

## CLEAN FIFTEEN™

| | | | |
|---|---|---|---|
| 1. | avocados | 9. | kiwis |
| 2. | sweet corn* | 10. | cabbages |
| 3. | pineapples | 11. | cauliflower |
| 4. | sweet peas (frozen) | 12. | cantaloupes |
| 5. | onions | 13. | broccoli |
| 6. | papayas* | 14. | mushrooms |
| 7. | eggplants | 15. | honeydew melons |
| 8. | asparagus | | |

* A small amount of sweet corn, papaya, and summer squash sold in the United States is produced from genetically modified seeds. Buy organic varieties of these crops if you want to avoid genetically modified produce.

# MEASUREMENT CONVERSIONS

## Volume Equivalents (Liquid)

| US STANDARD | US STANDARD (OUNCES) | METRIC (APPROXIMATE) |
|---|---|---|
| 2 tablespoons | 1 fl. oz. | 30 mL |
| ¼ cup | 2 fl. oz. | 60 mL |
| ½ cup | 4 fl. oz. | 120 mL |
| 1 cup | 8 fl. oz. | 240 mL |
| 1½ cups | 12 fl. oz. | 355 mL |
| 2 cups or 1 pint | 16 fl. oz. | 475 mL |
| 4 cups or 1 quart | 32 fl. oz. | 1 L |
| 1 gallon | 128 fl. oz. | 4 L |

## Volume Equivalents (Dry)

| US STANDARD | METRIC (APPROXIMATE) |
|---|---|
| ⅛ teaspoon | 0.5 mL |
| ¼ teaspoon | 1 mL |
| ½ teaspoon | 2 mL |
| ¾ teaspoon | 4 mL |
| 1 teaspoon | 5 mL |
| 1 tablespoon | 15 mL |
| ¼ cup | 59 mL |
| ⅓ cup | 79 mL |
| ½ cup | 118 mL |
| ⅔ cup | 156 mL |
| ¾ cup | 177 mL |
| 1 cup | 235 mL |
| 2 cups or 1 pint | 475 mL |
| 3 cups | 700 mL |
| 4 cups or 1 quart | 1 L |
| ½ gallon | 2 L |
| 1 gallon | 4 L |

## Oven Temperatures

| FAHRENHEIT (F) | CELSIUS (C) (APPROXIMATE) |
|---|---|
| 250°F | 120°C |
| 300°F | 150°C |
| 325°F | 165°C |
| 350°F | 180°C |
| 375°F | 190°C |
| 400°F | 200°C |
| 425°F | 220°C |
| 450°F | 230°C |

## Weight Equivalents

| US STANDARD | METRIC (APPROXIMATE) |
|---|---|
| ½ ounce | 15 g |
| 1 ounce | 30 g |
| 2 ounces | 60 g |
| 4 ounces | 115 g |
| 8 ounces | 225 g |
| 12 ounces | 340 g |
| 16 ounces or 1 pound | 455 g |

# RESOURCES

## Fertility and Pregnancy Supplements

All fertility supplements are not created equal, nor are all fertility supplements indicated for all people trying to conceive. Well Conceived Fertility provides a source of vetted, high-quality supplements for easier self-selection and peace of mind.

Well Conceived Fertility: wellconceivedfertility.com

## Fertility Self-Assessment

This fertility quiz is designed to help you identify where you're doing really well in your fertility journey, and where you can focus some additional support or self-care·

www.tworivershealth.ca/fertilityquiz

## Fish and Seafood

The following two resources can assist with shopping for more fertility- and pregnancy-safe fish choices:

EWG's Consumer Guide to Seafood: www.ewg.org/research/ewgs-good-seafood-guide

SeaChoice.org: www.seachoice.org

## Fertility Forums and Websites

There's no doubt that you'll want to find fertility related information online. I've found it's helpful to focus on sites that are vetted, positive, and that can offer a sense of connection with others who can understand what you're going through. Here are the three sites I recommend to my clients:

Fertility Matters: www.fertilitymatters.ca

Two Rivers Health: www.tworivershealth.ca/fertility

Fertility BoostCamp: www.facebook.com/groups /fertilityboostcamp

## Naturopathic Doctors In Your Area

American Association of Naturopathic Physicians (AANP): www.naturopathic.org

Canadian Association of Naturopathic Doctors (CAND): www.cand.ca

Ontario Association of Naturopathic Doctors (OAND): www.oand.org

## Fertility and Pregnancy Books

*8 Steps to Reverse Your PCOS*, by Dr. Fiona McCulloch, ND (2018)

*Fertility Secrets: What Your Doctor Didn't Tell You About Baby-Making*, by Dr. Aumatma Shah, ND (2017)

*Carrying to Term*, by Dr. Jordan Robertson, ND (2018)

*Real Food for Pregnancy*, by Lily Nichols, RDN, CDE (2017)

## Skin Care

These online resources make it easy to ensure that your daily skin care and cosmetics are fertility-friendly:

EWG Skin Deep Cosmetics Database: www.ewg.org/skindeep/
Natural Derm Store: www.NaturalDermStore.ca
The Truth Beauty Company: www.thetruthbeautycompany.com

## Water Filtration

By removing contaminants from your drinking water, you can reduce exposure to toxins that can negatively affect fertility and health. Availability of water filtration systems such as Berkey water filters or reverse osmosis installations will depend on where you live. In Canada and the United States, visit:

Canada:
http://www.consciouswater.ca/ref/wellconceived
United States:
www.berkeyfilters.com

# REFERENCES

## Chapter 1

ESHRE Capri Workshop Group. "Physiopathological Determinants of Human Infertility." *Human Reproduction Update* 8, no. 5 (2002): 435–447.

Ge, Z.J., Schatten, H., Zhang, C.L. and Sun, Q.Y. "Oocyte Ageing and Epigenetics." *Reproduction* (Cambridge, England) 149, no. 3 (2015): R103.

Haller-Kikkatalo, Kadri, Andres Salumets, and Raivo Uibo. "Review on Autoimmune Reactions in Female Infertility: Antibodies to Follicle Stimulating Hormone." *Clinical and Developmental Immunology* 2012 (2011).

Hunt, Patricia A., and Terry J. Hassold. "Human Female Meiosis: What Makes a Good Egg Go Bad?" *Trends in Genetics* 2 (2008): 86–93.

Khanna, Sunali Sundeep, Prita A. Dhaimade, and Shalini Malhotra. "Oral Health Status and Fertility Treatment Including IVF." *The Journal of Obstetrics and Gynecology of India* 67, no. 6 (2017): 400–404.

McCraty, Rollin, Bob Barrios-Choplin, Deborah Rozman, Mike Atkinson, and Alan D. Watkins. "The Impact of a New Emotional Self-Management Program on Stress, Emotions, Heart Rate Variability, DHEA and Cortisol." *Integrative Physiological and Behavioral Science* 33, no. 2 (1998): 151–170.

Simopoulou, M., et al. (2019). The Impact of Autoantibodies on IVF Treatment and Outcome: A Systematic Review. *International Journal of Molecular Sciences* 20, no. 4: 892. doi:10.3390/ijms20040892.

Steegers-Theunissen, Régine PM, John Twigt, Valerie Pestinger, and Kevin D. Sinclair. "The Periconceptional Period, Reproduction and Long-Term Health of Offspring: The Importance of One-Carbon Metabolism." *Human Reproduction Update* 19, no. 6 (2013): 640–655.

van den Boogaard, Emmy, Rosa Vissenberg, Jolande A. Land, Madelon van Wely, Joris AM van der Post, Mariette Goddijn, and Peter H. Bisschop. "Significance of (Sub) Clinical Thyroid Dysfunction and Thyroid Autoimmunity Before Conception and in Early Pregnancy: A Systematic Review." *Human Reproduction Update* 17, no. 5 (2011): 605–619.

Vujkovic, Marijana, Jeanne H. de Vries, Jan Lindemans, Nick S. Macklon, Peter J. van der Spek, Eric AP Steegers, and Régine PM Steegers-Theunissen. "The Preconception Mediterranean Dietary Pattern in Couples Undergoing In Vitro Fertilization/Intracytoplasmic Sperm Injection Treatment Increases the Chance of Pregnancy." *Fertility and Sterility* 94, no. 6 (2010): 2096–2101.

# Chapter 2

Akarsu, Süleyman, Funda Gode, Ahmet Zeki Isik, Zeliha Günnur Dikmen, and Mustafa Agah Tekindal. "The Association Between Coenzyme Q10 Concentrations in Follicular

Fluid with Embryo Morphokinetics and Pregnancy Rate in Assisted Reproductive Techniques." *Journal of Assisted Reproduction and Genetics* 34, no. 5 (2017): 599–605.

Bärebring, Linnea, Maria Bullarbo, Anna Glantz, Lena Hulthén, Joy Ellis, Åse Jagner, Inez Schoenmakers, Anna Winkvist, and Hanna Augustin. "Trajectory of Vitamin D Status During Pregnancy in Relation to Neonatal Birth Size and Fetal Survival: A Prospective Cohort Study." *BMC Pregnancy and Childbirth* 18, no. 1 (2018): 51.

Bevilacqua, Arturo, Gianfranco Carlomagno, Sandro Gerli, Mario Montanino Oliva, Paul Devroey, Antonio Lanzone, Christophe Soulange, et al. "Results From the International Consensus Conference on Myo-Inositol and D-Chiro-Inositol in Obstetrics and Gynecology–Assisted Reproduction Technology." *Gynecological Endocrinology* 31, no. 6 (2015): 441–446.

Briggs, D. A., D. J. Sharp, D. Miller, and R. G. Gosden. "Transferrin in the Developing Ovarian Follicle: Evidence for De-Novo Expression by Granulosa Cells." *MHR: Basic Science of Reproductive Medicine* 5, no. 12 (1999): 1107–1114.

Brouwer, Jenny, Johanna MW Hazes, Joop SE Laven, and Radboud JEM Dolhain. "Fertility in Women with Rheumatoid Arthritis: Influence of Disease Activity and Medication." *Annals of the Rheumatic Diseases* 74, no. 10 (2015): 1836–1841.

Casilla-Lennon, Marianne M., Samantha Meltzer-Brody, and Anne Z. Steiner. "The Effect of Antidepressants on

Fertility." *American Journal of Obstetrics and Gynecology* 215, no. 3 (2016): 314–e1.

Chavarro, Jorge E, Walter Willett, and Patrick J. Skerrett. *The Fertility Diet*. New York: McGraw Hill, 2009.

Clements Jr, Rex S., and Betty Darnell. "Myo-Inositol Content of Common Foods: Development of a High-Myo-Inositol Diet." *The American Journal of Clinical Nutrition* 33, no. 9 (1980): 1954–1967.

Croen, Lisa A., Judith K. Grether, Cathleen K. Yoshida, Roxana Odouli, and Victoria Hendrick. "Antidepressant Use During Pregnancy and Childhood Autism Spectrum Disorders." *Archives of General Psychiatry* 68, no. 11 (2011): 1104–1112.

Dell'Edera, D., F. Sarlo, A. Allegretti, A. A. Epifania, F. Simone, M. G. Lupo, M. Benedetto, M. R. D'APICE, and A. Capalbo. "Prevention of Neural Tube Defects and Maternal Gestational Diabetes Through the Inositol Supplementation: Preliminary Results." *European Review for Medical and Pharmacological Sciences* 21 (2017): 3305–3311.

Dolin, Cara D., Andrea L. Deierlein, and Mark I. Evans. "Folic Acid Supplementation to Prevent Recurrent Neural Tube Defects: 4 Milligrams Is Too Much." *Fetal Diagnosis and Therapy* 44, no. 3 (2018): 161–165.

Eke, A. C., G. Saccone, and V. Berghella. "Selective Serotonin Reuptake Inhibitor (SSRI) Use During Pregnancy and Risk of Preterm Birth: A Systematic Review and Meta-Analysis." *BJOG: An International Journal of Obstetrics & Gynecology* 123, no. 12 (2016): 1900–1907.

Environmental Working Group (EWG). "Dirty Dozen Endocrine Disruptors." 2013, www.ewg.org/research /dirty-dozen-list-endocrine-disruptors.

———"Exposures Add Up: Survey Results." 2019, www.ewg.org/ skindeep/2004/06/15/exposures-add-up-survey-results/

Giannubilo, Stefano, Patrick Orlando, Sonia Silvestri, Ilenia Cirilli, Fabio Marcheggiani, Andrea Ciavattini, and Luca Tiano. "CoQ10 Supplementation in Patients Undergoing IVF-ET: The Relationship with Follicular Fluid Content and Oocyte Maturity." *Antioxidants* 7, no. 10 (2018): 141.

Greenberg, James A., and Stacey J. Bell. "Multivitamin Supplementation During Pregnancy: Emphasis on Folic Acid and l-Methylfolate." *Reviews in Obstetrics and Gynecology* 4, no. 3–4 (2011): 126.

Health Canada. "Coenzyme Q10 (Ubiquinone-10)." 2018, webprod.hc-sc.gc.ca/nhpid-bdipsn/atReq.do?atid=coenzyme .q10&lang=eng.

Janssen, Namieta M., and Marcia S. Genta. "The Effects of Immunosuppressive and Anti-Inflammatory Medications on Fertility, Pregnancy, and Lactation." *Archives of Internal Medicine* 160, no. 5 (2000): 610–619.

Kalem, M. N., Z. Kalem, and T. Gurgan. "Effect of Metformin and Oral Contraceptives on Polycystic Ovary Syndrome and IVF Cycles." *Journal of Endocrinological Investigation* 40, no. 7 (2017): 745–752.

Kawachiya, Satoshi, Tsunekazu Matsumoto, Daniel Bodri, Keiichi Kato, Yuji Takehara, and Osamu Kato. "Short-Term, Low-Dose, Non-Steroidal Anti-Inflammatory Drug Application Diminishes Premature Ovulation in Natural-Cycle IVF." *Reproductive Biomedicine Online* 24, no. 3 (2012): 308–313.

Kolatorova, L., M. Duskova, J. Vitku, and L. Starka. "Prenatal Exposure to Bisphenols and Parabens and Impacts on Human Physiology." *Physiological Research* 66, no. 4 (2017).

Lamers, Yvonne, Amanda J. MacFarlane, Deborah L. O'Connor, and Bénédicte Fontaine-Bisson. "Periconceptional Intake of Folic Acid Among Low-Risk Women in Canada: Summary of a Workshop Aiming to Align Prenatal Folic Acid Supplement Composition with Current Expert Guidelines." *The American Journal of Clinical Nutrition* 108, no. 6 (2018): 1357–1368.

Leverrier-Penna, S., Mitchell, R.T., Becker, E., Lecante, L., Ben Maamar, M., Homer, N., Lavoué, V., Kristensen, D.M., Dejucq-Rainsford, N., Jégou, B. and Mazaud-Guittot, S. "Ibuprofen is Deleterious for the Development of First Trimester Human Fetal Ovary Ex Vivo." *Human Reproduction*, 33, no. 3 (2018): 482–493.

Li, Li, Xing Zhang, Lei Wang, Zhenhai Chai, Xiuping Shen, Zongpeng Zhang, and Changxiao Liu. "A Toxicology Study to Evaluate the Embryotoxicity of Metformin Compared with the Hypoglycemic Drugs, the Anticancer Drug, the Anti-Epileptic Drug, the Antibiotic, and the Cyclo-Oxygenase (COX)-2 Inhibitor." *Journal of Diabetes* 7, no. 6 (2015): 839–849.

Manfo, Faustin Pascal Tsagué, Rajamanickam Jubendradass, Edouard Akono Nantia, Paul Fewou Moundipa, and Premendu Prakash Mathur. "Adverse Effects of Bisphenol A on Male Reproductive Function." *Reviews of Environmental Contamination and Toxicology* 228 (2014): 57–82.

Matuszczak, Ewa, Marta Diana Komarowska, Wojciech Debek, and Adam Hermanowicz. "The Impact of Bisphenol A on Fertility, Reproductive System, and Development: A Review of the Literature." *International Journal of Endocrinology* (2019).

McCulloch, Fiona. *8 Steps to Reverse Your PCOS*. Austin, TX: Greenleaf Book Group, 2016.

Mok-Lin, E., S. Ehrlich, P. L. Williams, J. Petrozza, D. L. Wright, A. M. Calafat, X. Ye, and R. Hauser. "Urinary Bisphenol A Concentrations and Ovarian Response Among Women Undergoing IVF." *International Journal of Andrology* 33, no. 2 (2010): 385–393.

Polyzos, Nikolaos P., Ellen Anckaert, Luis Guzman, Johan Schiettecatte, Lisbet Van Landuyt, Michel Camus, Johan Smitz, and Herman Tournaye. "Vitamin D Deficiency and Pregnancy Rates in Women Undergoing Single Embryo, Blastocyst Stage, Transfer (SET) for IVF/ICSI." *Human Reproduction* 29, no. 9 (2014): 2032–2040.

Prasad, A. S., D. Oberleas, K. S. Moghissi, J. C. Stryker, and K. Y. Lei. "Effect of Oral Contraceptive Agents on Nutrients: II. Vitamins." *The American Journal of Clinical Nutrition* 28, no. 4 (1975): 385–391.

Quintino-Moro, Alessandra, Denise E. Zantut-Wittmann, Marcos Tambascia, Helymar da Costa Machado, and Arlete Fernandes. "High Prevalence of Infertility Among Women with Graves' Disease and Hashimoto's Thyroiditis." *International Journal of Endocrinology* 2014 (2014).

Regidor, Pedro-Antonio, Adolf Eduard Schindler, Bernd Lesoine, and Rene Druckman. "Management of Women with PCOS Using Myo-Inositol and Folic Acid. New Clinical Data and Review of the Literature." *Hormone Molecular Biology and Clinical Investigation* 34, no. 2 (2018).

Rochester, Johanna R. "Bisphenol A and Human Health: A Review of the Literature." *Reproductive Toxicology* 42 (2013): 132–155.

Simopoulou, Mara, Konstantinos Sfakianoudis, Evangelos Maziotis, Sokratis Grigoriadis, Polina Giannelou, Anna Rapani, Petroula Tsioulou, et al. "The Impact of Autoantibodies on IVF Treatment and Outcome: A Systematic Review." *International Journal of Molecular Sciences* 20, no. 4 (2019): 892.

Svirsky, Natali, Sigal Levy, and Ronit Avitsur. "Prenatal Exposure to Selective Serotonin Reuptake Inhibitors (SSRI) Increases Aggression and Modulates Maternal Behavior in Offspring Mice." *Developmental Psychobiology* 58, no. 1 (2016): 71–82.

Sylvester, Christie, Marie Menke, and Priya Gopalan. "Selective Serotonin Reuptake Inhibitors and Fertility:

Considerations for Couples Trying to Conceive." *Harvard Review of Psychiatry* 27, no. 2 (2019): 108–118.

Tiseo, Bruno C., Audrey J. Gaskins, Russ Hauser, Jorge E. Chavarro, Cigdem Tanrikut, and EARTH Study Team. "Coenzyme Q10 Intake from Food and Semen Parameters in a Subfertile Population." *Urology* 102 (2017): 100–105.

Tomioka, Renato B., Gabriela RV Ferreira, Nadia E. Aikawa, Gustavo AR Maciel, Paulo C. Serafini, Adriana M. Sallum, Lucia MA Campos, Claudia Goldestein-Schainberg, Eloisa Bonfá, and Clovis A. Silva. "Non-Steroidal Anti-Inflammatory Drug Induces Luteinized Unruptured Follicle Syndrome in Young Female Juvenile Idiopathic Arthritis Patients." *Clinical Rheumatology* 37, no. 10 (2018): 2869–2873.

Turi, Angelo, Stefano Raffaele Giannubilo, Francesca Brugè, Federica Principi, Silvia Battistoni, Fabrizia Santoni, Andrea Luigi Tranquilli, GianPaolo Littarru, and Luca Tiano. "Coenzyme Q10 Content in Follicular Fluid and Its Relationship with Oocyte Fertilization and Embryo Grading." *Archives of Gynecology and Obstetrics* 285, no. 4 (2012): 1173–1176.

USDA. "USDA Food Composition Databases." 2018, ndb.nal .usda.gov/ndb/.

Wilson, R. Douglas, François Audibert, Jo-Ann Brock, June Carroll, Lola Cartier, Alain Gagnon, Jo-Ann Johnson et al. "Pre-Conception Folic Acid and Multivitamin Supplementation for the Primary and Secondary Prevention of Neural Tube Defects and Other Folic Acid-Sensitive Congenital

Anomalies." *Journal of Obstetrics and Gynaecology Canada* 37, no. 6 (2015): 534–549.

Yu, Weonjin, Yi-Chun Yen, Young-Hwan Lee, Shawn Tan, Yixin Xiao, Hidayat Lokman, Audrey Khoo Tze Ting et al. "Prenatal Selective Serotonin Reuptake Inhibitor (SSRI) Exposure Induces Working Memory and Social Recognition Deficits by Disrupting Inhibitory Synaptic Networks in Male Mice." *Molecular Brain* 12, no. 1 (2019): 29.

Zheng, Xiangqin, Danmei Lin, Yulong Zhang, Yuan Lin, Jianrong Song, Suyu Li, and Yan Sun. "Inositol Supplement Improves Clinical Pregnancy Rate in Infertile Women Undergoing Ovulation Induction for ICSI or IVF-ET." *Medicine* 96, no. 49 (2017).

# Chapter 3

Chavarro, Jorge E, Walter Willett, and Patrick J. Skerrett. *The Fertility Diet.* New York: McGraw Hill, 2009.

Harb, H. M., I.D. Gallos, J. Chu, M. Harb, and A. Coomarasamy. "The Effect of Endometriosis on in Vitro Fertilisation Outcome: A Systematic Review and Meta-Analysis." *BJOG: An International Journal of Obstetrics & Gynaecology* 120, no. 11 (2013): 1308–1320.

Jakubowicz, Daniela, Maayan Barnea, Julio Wainstein, and Oren Froy. "Effects of Caloric Intake Timing on Insulin Resistance and Hyperandrogenism in Lean Women with Polycystic Ovary Syndrome." *Clinical Science* 125, no. 9 (2013): 423–432.

Máté, Gábor, Lori Robin Bernstein, and Attila Laszlo Torok. "Endometriosis is a Cause of Infertility. Does Reactive Oxygen Damage to Gametes and Embryos Play a Key Role in the Pathogenesis of Infertility Caused by Endometriosis?" *Frontiers in Endocrinology* 9 (2018): 725.

McCulloch, Fiona. *8 Steps to Reverse Your PCOS*. Austin, TX: 2016. Greenleaf Book Group, 2016.

Vujkovic, Marijana, Jeanne H. de Vries, Jan Lindemans, Nick S. Macklon, Peter J. van der Spek, Eric AP Steegers, and Régine PM Steegers-Theunissen. "The Preconception Mediterranean Dietary Pattern in Couples Undergoing In Vitro Fertilization/Intracytoplasmic Sperm Injection Treatment Increases the Chance of Pregnancy." *Fertility and Sterility* 94, no. 6 (2010): 2096–2101.

# INDEX

# ACKNOWLEDGMENTS

I'd like to thank Callisto Media for the opportunity and support in publishing this book (my first!), especially Morgan Shanahan and Claire Yee for your editorial guidance with the manuscript. Thank you to my friend, chef Charleston Dollano, for the creative, delicious, and nourishing recipes; I couldn't have done this without you!

I also want to thank my sister, Stephanie Vandekemp, for always inspiring me to take on the next adventure, my husband for believing in my ability to bring this labor of love into the world, and my friends, family, and team at Two Rivers Health for encouraging me.

Most of all, thank you to my patients and clients for being the truest source of inspiration for this book. You've taught me more about healing, humanity, and creating our own definitions of "having it all" than I ever could have imagined. It's been a long time since some of you began encouraging me to write a book, and I deeply appreciate the privilege of walking alongside you on your paths to parenthood and beyond. I respect the work we do together as life-changing, miraculous, and our gift to the next generation. Thank you.

# ABOUT THE AUTHOR

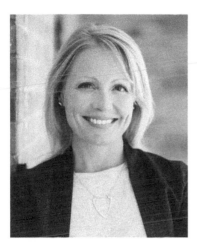

**Dr. Elizabeth Cherevaty, ND, RAC,** is a naturopathic doctor with a special focus in integrative fertility, women's and children's health, and feminine leadership. As the founding director of Two Rivers Health, she created the Well Conceived Fertility Method™, an evidence-based program dedicated to helping women and couples build their fertile foundations, break through obstacles to pregnancy, and bring their healthy, happy babies home.

She's passionate about inspiring women globally to embrace their feminine power, so they can create their own definitions of "having it all."

Dr. Cherevaty invites women who are seeking support with their fertility journey to book a complimentary Conception Confidence Call through her clinic website.

Website: www.tworivershealth.ca
Facebook: www.facebook.com/groups/fertilityboostcamp
Instagram: @elizabeth.cherevaty

# ABOUT THE RECIPE DEVELOPER

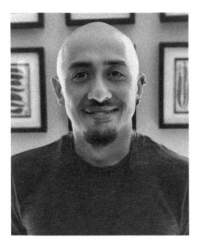

**Charleston F. Dollano** is a chef and educator. His ambition and philosophy is to educate people about the joys of eating whole foods, support sustainable agriculture, and bridge the gap between the farm and the table. He encourages cooks to exercise their creativity in the kitchen by adjusting recipes to their individual palates and preferences. Together with his wife, Katrina, the Chinese medicine practitioner at What's Good, Charleston aims to combine traditional Chinese medicine dietetics with modern food trends to create nutritional, healing meals that address patients' dietary needs, including helping women and couples conceive and have healthy pregnancies. When Charleston is not cooking, he enjoys dancing, snowboarding, grocery shopping, and writing about himself in the third person.

Website: www.whatsgoodwellness.ca
Facebook: www.facebook.com/whatsgoodwellness
Instagram: @whatsgoodwellness